How To Make Authentic English Recipes

The Complete 10 Volume Set

✍

Geoff Wells

Authentic English Recipes
Book 11

Copyright© 2018 by Geoff Wells

All rights reserved

No part of this book may be used or reproduced in any manner whatsoever without prior written permission from the publisher, except for the inclusion of brief quotations in reviews.

Cover Artwork & Design by
Old Geezer Designs

Published in the United States by
Authentic English Recipes
an imprint of
DataIsland Software LLC,
Hollywood, Florida

https://ebooks.geezerguides.com

ISBN-13: 978-1479336586

ISBN-10: 1479336580

Neither the author nor the publisher assumes responsibility for errors in internet addresses or for changes in the addresses after publication. Nor are they responsible for the content of websites they do not own.

Table of Contents

DEDICATION

AIR FRYER & INSTANT POT METHODS 1

FISH & CHIPS 2

INTRODUCTION 3
   What Does Authentic Mean? 3

INGREDIENTS 4
   Chips 4
   Fish 4
   Get It Fresh 4
   Or Frozen 5
   The Oil 5
   Cooking In Oil 6
   Mushy Peas 6

MAKE IT CONVENIENT 7
   Wrapping It Up 7

MY PERSONAL BEER BATTER RECIPE 8

RECAP: AUTHENTIC ENGLISH FISH & CHIPS 9
   Chips 9
   Fish 9
   Batter 9
   Oil 9
   Cook 10
   Serve 10
   Pre-cook for Deep Frying Later 10
   Newspaper 10

AIR FRYER CHIPS
(FRENCH FRIES) 11

AIR FRYER FROZEN BATTERED FISH 13

Sherry Trifle 14

Is There Any Such Thing As Authentic English Trifle? 15
- The Bowl 15
- Trifle Bottom 16
- My Way 16
- Traditional Additions 18

Toppings 19
- Birds Custard 19
- Real Whipped Cream 19

Making Real Whipped Cream 20
- Substitute Custard 20

Trifle Recap 22

Fools 23

Gooseberry Fool 24

Blackberry Fool 25

Rhubarb Fool 26

Strawberry Fool 27

Strawberry Rhubarb Fool 28

Raspberry Fool 29

BONUS! - Raspberry Hack 30

Mango Fool 31

Beef Stew 32

How to Make a Perfect Stew Every Time 33
- Rule #5 Taste It Before You Serve It 33

Stock 34

SPLIT PEAS 36
   Yellow Split Peas Pudding 36

RECIPES 37

VEGETABLES 38

SPICES 39
   Bouillon 39
   Salt 39

THE PROCESS 40
   Prepare Your Vegetables 40

THICKENING 41

LEFTOVER STEW 42

A WORD ABOUT DUMPLINGS 43

SUET DUMPLINGS 44

WHEN IT ALL GOES PEAR-SHAPED 45
   Too Thick 45
   Too Thin 45
   No Taste 45
   Too Salty 45

BEST BEEF STEW EVER 46
   The Beef 46
   Kidney 46
   Sear the Meat 47
   Add Water 47
   Add Vegetables 47
   Bovril™ 47
   Cook Slowly 47
   Taste It 47
   Thicken It 48
   Let The Flavors Mature 48
   Steak And Kidney Pie 48

RECIPE RECAP 49

INSTANT POT - BEST BEEF STEW EVER 50

LIVER & ONIONS 51

GOURMET STYLE LIVER AND ONIONS DINNER 52

LIVER 53

BACON 54
English Bacon 54
American Bacon 54
Canadian Bacon 54
Which Bacon To Use? 54
Dripping 54

SPINACH 55
Baby Spinach 55
Regular Spinach 55
Cooking Spinach 55

ADDITIONAL INGREDIENTS 56
Onion 56
Tip 56
Whipped Potatoes 56
How much salt? 56
Tip 56
Colemans™ Mustard 57

PUTTING IT ALL TOGETHER 58
Step 1 - The Bacon 58
Step 2 - The Onion 58
Step 3 - The Potatoes 58
Step 4 - The Spinach 59
Step 5 - The Liver 59
Step 6 - The Gravy 59
Step 7 - Whip the Potatoes 60
Step 8 - Plate It 60

Wine	60

Recap 61
Bacon	61
Potatoes and Spinach	61
Liver	61
Gravy	62
Colemans™ Mustard	62
Plating	62

Instant Pot™ Mashed Potatoes 63

Sunday Roast 64

The Sunday Roast 65
Selecting the meat.	65
Lamb	65
Pork	65
Beef	65
How To Roast	66

Oven Roasting Beef 67
Seasoning	67
Searing	67
Beef Cooking Times	67

Oven Roasting Lamb 68
Seasoning	68
Searing	68
Lamb Cooking Times	68

Oven Roasting Pork 69
Seasoning	69
Searing	69
Pork Cooking Times	69

Oven Roasting Poultry 70
Seasoning	70
Searing	70

Poultry Cooking Times 70

CONDIMENTS 71
Mint Sauce (For Lamb) 71
AppleSauce (For Pork) 71
Horseradish Sauce (For Beef) 71
Sage & Onion Stuffing (For Poultry) 72

STUFFING BREAD 73

SAGE & ONION STUFFING 74

YORKSHIRE PUDDING 75
Success Is In The Details 76
Salt 76
Rest 76
Cook It 76
Two Ways 77

ROAST POTATOES & PARSNIPS 78
Crispy Roast Potatoes & Parsnips 78
Pan Roasted Potatoes & Parsnips 79
Air Fryer Roast Potatoes & Parsnips 79

ONION SAUCE 80

GREEN VEG & CARROTS 81
Steaming 81
Scarlet Runner Beans 81
Carrots 81

GRAVY 82

DESSERT 83

AND NOW FOR SOMETHING COMPLETELY DIFFERENT - PANCAKES (CRÊPES) 84

TOAD IN THE HOLE 85

INSTANT POT ROASTING 86

Air Fryer
Roast Potatoes and Parsnips 88

Instant Pot Applesauce 90

English Breakfast 91

How To Make An English Breakfast 92

Traditional English-Style Baked Beans 95

Homemade Baked Beans With molasses 96

English Breakfast
Recipe Recap 97

A Lighter British Breakfast 99

English Muffins 100

Poached Eggs on an English Muffin 102

Instant Pot Traditional English-Style
Baked Beans (No-soak method) 103

Instant Pot Homemade Baked Beans
With Molasses 105

Instant Pot Poached Eggs 106

Instant Pot
Almond Buckwheat Porridge 107

Instant Pot
Apple and Spice Steel Cut Oats 108

Devonshire Tea 109

Introduction 110

How to Make Real English Tea 111
  Real Tea 111
  Tea Bags 111
  Tea Balls 111

Making a Cuppa ... 112
Boiling Water ... 112
Warm the Pot ... 112
Add the Tea ... 112
Bring the Teapot to the Kettle ... 112
Steep It ... 112
Milk, Sugar or Lemon ... 112
Recap ... 113

How To Make Scones ... 114

How To Make Strawberry Jam ... 115

How To Make Clotted Cream ... 116
Serving ... 117

Instant Pot Strawberry Jam ... 118

Instant Pot Clotted Cream ... 119

Whey Scones ... 120

Cornish Pasties ... 121

Introduction ... 122
The Protected Pasty ... 122

Cornish Pasty Association ... 123

The Official Cornish Pasty Recipe ... 124

The Official Cornish Pasty ~ US Version ... 126

Flaky Pastry Recipe ... 128

Unofficial Cornish Pasty Appetizers ... 129

Savory Pasties ... 131

Vegetarian Pasty ... 132

Cheese, Mushroom and Leek ... 133

Ham, Swiss Cheese and Asparagus ... 134

Sausage Pasty 135

Pizza Pasty 136

Asian Pasty 137

Jerk Chicken Pasty 138

Dessert Pasties 139

Peach & Walnut Pasty 140

Bumbleberry Pasties 141

Banana & Chocolate Pasty 142

Banana Split Pasty 143

Apple and Walnut Pasty 144

Instant Pot Cornish Pasty
Appetizers Filling 145

British Cakes 146

Introduction 147

Bakewell Tarts 148
 To make the icing 149

English Shortbread 150

Scones 151

Chelsea Buns 152

Chelsea Buns
(Bread Machine Method) 154
 To make the glaze 155

Victoria Sponge Cake 156
 Whip The Cream 157

Crumpets 158

CRUMPETS
(BREAD MACHINE METHOD) 160

CUSTARD TARTS 161
  Variations 162

DUNDEE CAKE 163

ENGLISH BATH BUNS
(BREAD MACHINE METHOD) 165

ENGLISH MUFFINS 167

ENGLISH MUFFINS
(BREAD MACHINE METHOD) 169

DIGESTIVE BISCUITS 171

HOT CROSS BUNS (BREAD MACHINE METHOD) 173
  Making the Pastry Crosses 174
  Making the Egg Wash 174
  Glazing the Buns 175

MADELEINES 176

MAID OF HONOUR TARTS 178

SAUSAGE ROLLS 179

PASTRY TART SHELLS 180

INSTANT POT DUNDEE CAKE 181

AIR FRYER SAUSAGE ROLLS 183

SPOTTED DICK 184

INTRODUCTION 185
  FAQ's 186
    What Is Suet? 186
    Where Can I Buy Suet? 186
    From The Butcher 186

Substitutes for Suet 186
What Is A Steamed Pudding? 187
What's A Pudding Cloth? 187
What Is A Pudding Basin? 187
Must I Use A Pudding Basin? 188
How Much Cooking Water Do I Use? 188
Self-Raising Flour 188
Measuring Ingredients 188

Basic Suet Crust 189
A Few Tips 189
How To Steam 189
Using A Steamer 189
Using an Instant Pot 190

Savoury Suet Pastry 191

Sweet Suet Pastry 192

Spotted Dick 193

Suet Dumplings 195
Suggestions 195

Apple and Blackberry Suet Pudding 196
Suggestions 196

Carrot-Raisin Suet Pudding 197

Christmas Plum Pudding 198

Figgy Pudding 200

Ginger Pudding 202

Jam Roly-Poly 203
Baked Roly-Poly 203

Leicestershire Pudding 204

Lemony Sussex Pond Pudding 205

MIDDLESEX POND PUDDING 206
TREACLE PUDDING 208
BONUS RECIPE - MINCEMEAT 209
CHEESE AND LEEK SUET PUDDING 210
HAM AND LEEK SUET PUDDING 211
STEAK AND KIDNEY PUDDING.. 212
INSTANT POT STEAMED PUDDINGS................................. 214
INSTANT POT SPOTTED DICK 215
INSTANT POT APPLE AND BLACKBERRY PUDDING 217
INSTANT POT CARROT-RAISIN PUDDING 219
INSTANT POT CHRISTMAS PLUM PUDDING 221
INSTANT POT FIGGY PUDDING 224
INSTANT POT GINGER PUDDING 226
INSTANT POT JAM ROLY-POLY....................................... 228
INSTANT POT LEICESTERSHIRE PUDDING 229
INSTANT POT LEMONY SUSSEX POND PUDDING............ 231
INSTANT POT MIDDLESEX POND PUDDING 233
INSTANT POT TREACLE PUDDING 235
INSTANT POT CHEESE AND LEEK SUET PUDDING 237
INSTANT POT HAM AND LEEK SUET PUDDING 239
INSTANT POT STEAK AND KIDNEY PUDDING................. 241

EXTRA SPECIAL BONUS............................ 244

MOM'S GREEN TOMATO CHUTNEY
INSTANT POT VERSION 246

BONUS ~ Claim Your Free Book 247
About The Author 248
About Our Cookbooks 249
　Quality 249
　Consistency 249
　Only Quality Ingredients 249
　English Speaking Authors 249
　Found an Error? 249
Published by Geezer Guides 250

Dedication

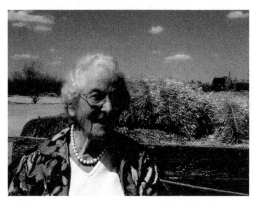

This series of books are dedicated to Mildred Ellen Wells 1906 - 2008

Mom lived for 102 incredible years. She went from horse drawn carriages and sailing ships to bullet trains and moon rockets.

She was not a fancy cook but everything she made tasted great. My dad grew much of what we ate in our garden so everything was always fresh and free of chemicals.

This book is a collection of some of her best recipes. I have just translated the quantities for the North American market.

I know she would be delighted to see all her recipes collected together so that you can continue to make these great tasting dishes.

Geoff Wells - Ontario, Canada - September 2012

Air Fryer & Instant Pot Methods

I guess when it comes to these new fangled gadgets, we're a little late to the party, but they have now found an important place in our kitchen.

We use these new appliances so much we decided to re-release the Authentic English Recipes series with Air Fryer and Instant Pot directions for all appropriate recipes.

We have also added videos for all these recipes to our

<https://instantpotvideorecipes.com>

membership site.

As one of our loyal readers you get a free membership to this site as a bonus for buying this book. All you do is visit the secret claim page to get your 100% discount coupon code.

<https://fun.geezerguides.com/freemembership>

Fish & Chips

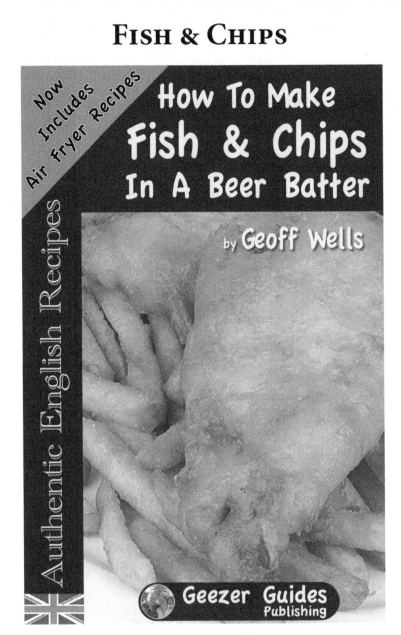

Introduction

What Does Authentic Mean?

The signs proclaim "Authentic English Fish and Chips" in two foot high flashing neon lights but what they serve is fish fingers with shoestring fries. Trust me, that's not authentic. I even had fish and chips in Phoenix, Arizona where the batter was made from corn meal.

You have a better chance of finding an honest politician in Washington, DC than finding authentic fish and chips in America.

What does that mean anyway? What is authentic English fish and chips?

Even in England the fish and chips range from mediocre to outstanding. At least you will never get a corn meal batter - Ugh!

When I was growing up in England we had access to at least three fish and chip shops (local chippies) within easy walking distance of our house.

Our favorite shop was next door to the Flying Eagle Pub. It's gone now and the Flying Eagle has become an Indian restaurant. But I still fondly remember picking up six-pennyworth of chips as I walked home from school.

Ingredients

Chips

If you want authentic, you need to start with the chips. They should be hand cut, then soaked in salted water for an hour or so to get the starch out. They must not be the awful shoestring fries that are cold before you even have a chance to eat them. Proper chips, for your authentic fish and chip dinner, are thick, crisp and golden brown.

After you have soaked them in the salted water, drain them completely and then pat them dry with paper towel. In my restaurant I used to lightly pre-cook them so my customers didn't have to wait forever for their order, because fish cooks a lot quicker than raw potato.

The potatoes are usually peeled, of course, but personally I prefer to leave the skin on. It's less "authentic" but I don't care.

Fish

The choice of fish at our local chippy was usually cod, haddock, skate and rock salmon.

My personal favorite was rock salmon, also called rock eel or dogfish. I can hear all the Americans going "Eel! Ugh!" But it was wonderful and it was what I was brought up with so I never questioned it. Actually it is a small shark that has been overfished and is now threatened with extinction so obviously it's not available anymore.

Cod was our next choice although I liked haddock better. But in my youth haddock was a more expensive option, so we usually had the cod. I really don't remember ever having skate - I guess my parents didn't like it.

Get It Fresh

But all these authentic fish had been swimming in the ocean just the day before we ate them. Early every morning fishmongers would make the trip to Billingsgate Fish Market in London to purchase their supplies for the day and I don't think that has changed to this day. England is a very small island with a rich fishing tradition, so fresh fish is something we took for granted.

In North America because of the size of the country the places to find fresh fish are very limited, unless you catch your own or live along a coast. Most likely you will head to the supermarket to get your fish and end up buying some frozen, pre-battered piece of tilapia in a boil-in bag - Ugh!

Or Frozen

All is not lost. You can buy some decent frozen fish in the supermarket. In Canada we get the "Highliner™" brand that has fish fillet blocks about 9 inches long x 3 inches wide and ½ inches thick. You can get cod, haddock, Boston blue and probably tilapia. Tilapia has the distinction of being the only fish with a total absence of flavor. When cooked it shrinks to half its size and has the texture of wet cardboard. Can you tell I'm not a big fan?

When shopping for your fish look for a real fillet of haddock or Boston blue. No, Boston blue is not authentic because they don't catch that in England, but it is a very nice fish and it is what I served in my restaurant.

The Oil

You can make passable chips in a frying pan or even healthier versions by tossing them in oil and baking them in an oven, but battered fish must be deep-fried.

You can deep-fry your battered fish in a pot of oil on the stove but it makes quite a fire hazard and a real mess if you drop it. That's a childhood trauma I won't soon forget. There was grease everywhere. Boy did I get heck!

A better option is to buy an electric countertop deep fryer at Wal-Mart, or from Amazon, for about $25 to $50, which does an excellent job for a small family. These small deep fryers don't hold much so you should plan to cook at least a couple of batches.

If you have an Air Fryer you can get excellent results with hardly any oil. See the Air Fryer section later in this book.

It's important to use a good quality oil that can stand up to high temperatures. Peanut oil is a good choice. If you're allergic to peanuts, then safflower or sunflower oil are good options. Canola oil has a lower smoke point but is still okay. Olive oil is not a good choice for this type of cooking because it is likely to smoke at deep frying temperatures.

Make sure that your fish is fully defrosted and patted dry with paper towel before your try to batter it.

The Batter

Put your batter in a long, shallow dish to make the battering process easier. A loaf pan or similar type of dish will work.

Yes, I'm going to give you my personal beer batter recipe at the end of the book, but read on so that you'll have all the information you need before you make your first batch.

The batter needs to be thick enough that it will stick to the fish without dripping into the oil too much.

Put the fish in the batter and make sure it is completely covered. Pick up the fish and let the excess batter drain back into the dish.

COOKING IN OIL

Lower the fish slowly into the hot oil (375°F or 190°C). Be careful not to drop it because you don't want to splash the hot oil. When the batter is golden brown, the fish is done. Most kinds of fish cook very quickly and you don't want to over cook it.

The chips are going to take much longer to cook than the fish, so you should cook them first. If you have a large enough fry basket you can add the fish when the chips start to change color. Odds are, though, that you'll have to cook the chips separately from the fish. Transfer the chips to a separate dish and keep them warm in the oven until the fish is ready.

Before putting your hand cut chips into the hot oil, make sure they are reasonably dry. Any excess water will cause the oil to spit and you could burn yourself. Excess water in the oil will also shorten the number of times you can re-use the oil.

MUSHY PEAS

It seems that an authentic English fish and chips dinner now includes mushy peas. This was not true when I was growing up in London, but now it seems to be widespread. Mushy peas used to be a strictly Northern England thing but maybe Coronation Street fever took over as that's what they'd serve with fish and chips at Rovers Return. We like fresh or frozen peas with our fish and chips and are not fans of mushy peas. Basically they are marrowfat peas that are soaked overnight in water and then simmered with a little sugar and salt until they form a thick, green, lumpy soup.

MAKE IT CONVENIENT

I used to own a restaurant in a tourist area not far from Toronto, Canada. We sold a lot of fish and chips along with a lot of other dishes as well. The batter for the fish was often a problem because it was frequently in the way and, when we got really busy, I would run out of batter and have to stop to make more. The solution was to pre-batter the fish, pre-cook it slightly and then freeze it. All you need to do is to batter the fish in the regular way and then pop it in the hot oil for just a few seconds (10 - 15). That's just long enough to set the batter. Wrap each slightly pre-cooked piece individually and then freeze them. This makes it really convenient when you want some fish and chips because now you don't have to mess around with the batter. The fish is ready to go into the hot oil, right from the freezer. Gently put the frozen, pre-battered fish into the hot oil, just like you would freshly battered fish, and when it's golden brown, it's done.

WRAPPING IT UP

A popular misconception is that in England fish and chips comes wrapped in newspaper - and nothing else. Layers of newspaper is a great insulator and so the package is usually outer wrapped in newspaper which keeps it warm until you get it home. You can trust that your food is in a box or grease proof bag and is quite sanitary.

SERVE

Shake some salt on both the fish and the chips then add malt vinegar. Malt vinegar is another one of those things you have to search for in North America. It is still available and the effort of finding it is well worth it.

Every fish and chip shop always had a big jar of pickled onions on the counter. If you can find them in your supermarket pick up a jar - or two.

My Personal Beer Batter Recipe

Here's my personal beer batter recipe. The beer adds flavor but, most importantly, the carbonation makes it light and crispy.

I suppose you could substitute soda water if you object to the beer. Maybe even 7-Up for a lemon/lime flavor. The downside of using pop/soda, of course, is that you are adding a massive amount of sugar to your diet.

I've never tried it so there's no guarantee. Please let me know if you do.

Ingredients

    2 cups (240g) all-purpose flour
    ½ oz. (1½ tablespoons, 22mL) dry active yeast
    16 oz.(2 cups, 475mL) beer
    2 tablespoons (30 mL) vegetable oil (I use peanut oil)
    1 egg white

Method

Combine first four ingredients - flour, yeast, beer, vegetable oil - and mix well.

Cover with a damp cloth and let stand for 10 minutes.

At the last moment, just before use, mix in the egg white.

Recap: Authentic English Fish & Chips

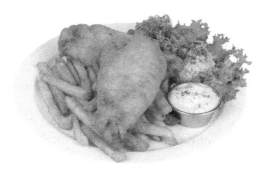

Chips

Hand cut your chips from real potatoes. They should be chunky, not shoestring-type potatoes.

Soak the chips in salted water for about an hour. Drain off the water and pat-dry the chips with paper towels.

Cook the chips first, as they take a lot longer to cook than the fish does. Deep fry the chips until they are a nice golden brown. If necessary place them in a separate dish and keep them warm in the oven while you cook the fish.

Alternately, you can fry the chips in a frying pan on top of the stove, or toss them in oil and bake them in a hot oven (425°F or 220°C) for about 20-30 minutes depending on their thickness, turning once about halfway through. Oven fries are in no way authentic but they are slightly better for you.

Fish

Make sure your fish is completely thawed (if using frozen fish), then pat the fish dry so that the batter will stick properly.

Batter

Prepare your batter using the recipe above.

Place the batter in a shallow dish to make it easy to batter the fish.

Place the fish in that batter and make sure it is totally covered. Lift the fish out of the batter and let any excess batter drip back into the dish.

Oil

The best oils for deep frying are peanut oil, safflower oil, sunflower oil or canola oil, in that order. Olive oil will smoke at frying temperature.

Preheat the oil in your deep fryer to 375°F (190°C).

Cook

When the oil is ready, gently lower the battered fish into the hot oil. Be careful not to drop it.

When the batter is golden brown, the fish is ready. Remove it from the deep fryer letting any excess oil drain off.

Serve

Serve with fresh peas (mushy if you must), salt and malt vinegar. Maybe a pickled onion . You'll never find tarter sauce in a local chippie.

Pre-cook for Deep Frying Later

If you want to freeze some of the battered fish to deep fry, directly from frozen, later, follow the instructions above, with one exception. Deep fry the battered fish for about 10-15 seconds. That's just enough time to set the batter.

Let the slightly pre-cooked fish cool on some paper towel and then wrap each piece individually in plastic wrap and freeze for later use.

Newspaper

Optional

Air Fryer Chips
(French Fries)

Air frying times and temperatures will vary depending on the size of the fries and amount.

This recipe will give you a good rule of thumb.

Note

1. Be sure to use either Russet or Yukon Gold potatoes as they work best and make tasty chips.

2. Most recipes will tell you to peel the potatoes, I don't Why? - For a couple of reasons:

a) There's really no need to; most of the nutrition is in the peel, so why waste it;

b) I think they taste better with the skins left on.

Ingredients

3 to 4 medium Russet or Yukon Gold potatoes, scrubbed
1 Tablespoon (15 mL) extra virgin olive oil
Sea salt or Himalayan pink salt

Directions

1. Cut the well scrubbed potatoes into ½ inch (1.25 cm) strips or in wedges if you desire (wedges will take a little longer to cook).
2. Soak the cut potatoes in cold water for at least ½ hour.
3. Drain the potatoes and dry them thoroughly.
4. Pre-heat the air fryer to 375-400° F (190-200°C). Use the lower temperature for thinner chips, the higher temperature for larger chips or wedges.
5. Place the chips in a shallow bowl and drizzle them with the olive oil. Then toss to make sure all the chips are evenly coated. Optionally, you can spray the chips with olive oil using a mister. We use the Misto which you can pick up on Amazon at http://amzn.to/2sdcOWI

6. Place the chips (or wedges) in the basket and cook for 10 minutes.
7. Remove the basket. Shake well. Return the basket to the air fryer and cook for an additional 10 minutes.
8. Season with salt and serve.

Note: If you plan to do both the chips and the fish in your air fryer, cook the chips first and keep them warm in your oven at about 170° F (75° C).

Air Fryer Frozen Battered Fish

Although it would be nice to cook the fish from fresh in an air fryer, that's just not possible. The fan on an air fryer will blow the batter off before it has a chance to set. But that doesn't mean you can't use your air fryer to make fish & chips.

I had a similar problem in my restaurant. My fish and chips were very popular but they were not the only thing on the menu and the batter makes a mess of the deep fryer. Also, cooking the fish fresh would mean having a bowl of batter around all the time.

The secret to solving this problem is to batter your fillets in batches and fry them just enough to set the batter. Then, after they cool wrap them up and freeze them.

You can use these partially cooked, frozen fillets in the air fryer without worrying about spraying batter. If you keep a few of these battered fillets in the freezer you'll be able to have fresh cooked fish and chips any time you want.

Ingredients

2-3 partially cooked, battered fish fillets (how many will fit in the air fryer basket will depend on the size of each fillet)
Extra virgin olive oil

Directions

1. Pre-heat the air fryer to 400° F (200° C).
2. Using a pastry brush, brush the battered fillets with the olive oil on both sides. Optionally, you can spray the fillets with olive oil using a mister. We use the Misto which you can pick up on Amazon at http://amzn.to/2sdcOWI
3. Place 2 or 3 (depending on size) of the frozen fillets in the basket all in one layer and cook for 8-10 minutes (depending on size and thickness).
4. Remove the basket, gently turn the fillets and return the basket to the air fryer.
5. Cook for another 8-10 minutes. You might need to increase this time for thicker or larger fillets, but they should be nicely browned and crisp.
6. Remove fillets from basket and serve.

Note: If you plan to do both the chips and the fish in your air fryer, cook the chips first and keep them warm in your oven at about 170° F (75° C).

Sherry Trifle

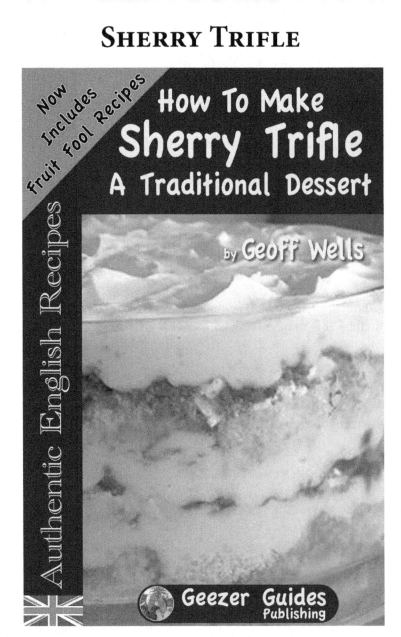

Is There Any Such Thing As Authentic English Trifle?

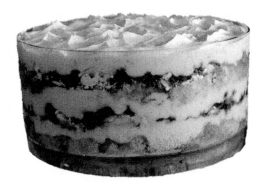

Not really - kind of - maybe. The problem is that everyone - even in England - has their own idea of how to make "real" trifle. There are, at least, a few common ideas about what a real trifle contains. Maybe not ingredients, exactly, but at least a sort of structure.

Let's start with the basics. We all agree it's a dessert. It has a sort of cakey base, fruit, custard and whipped cream. Beyond that it's anybody's guess what you will be served when you order "authentic" English trifle.

Growing up in England, I didn't know there could be so many versions of something I thought of as a staple. As far as I knew, my mother's trifle was the definitive dessert that was served for all special occasions, like birthdays and Christmas.

Fortunately for you, since I will be sharing this recipe in a moment, my mother's trifle is the best trifle recipe you will ever find. I say that with the authority of sampling other trifles for more than 50 years across England and North America.

To be fair to my American friends, there are some ingredients that are difficult, if not impossible, to buy in American supermarkets. Don't worry, I'll offer some alternatives as we get to them.

The Bowl

Trifle is made in a large bowl. You can actually buy a "trifle bowl" quite easily from Amazon or Bed, Bath & Beyond. The ones I see online look a little small, but it doesn't matter as this "recipe" is more about the ingredients and the procedure than it is about quantities.

With the right trifle bowl a trifle is as much a feast for the eyes as it for the taste buds. A trifle bowl is made of glass, has a pedestal base and deep straight sides. Just Google trifle bowl images and you will see just how good they look.

Don't put off making a trifle just because you don't have the right bowl - it will taste just as good no matter what you make it in. But for a dinner party a properly prepared trifle in a traditional trifle bowl makes a spectacular presentation.

Trifle Bottom

Most recipes I see call for some sort of sponge or pound cake as a base. It will work okay and I have used a plain cake myself a few times but the preferred base is ladyfinger biscuits. These are a recognized type of biscuit (try Google) and are available worldwide. They usually come in cellophane packages and you will need 3 or 4 packages depending on the size of your trifle bowl.

Your trifle is going to be made with layers of ladyfingers and fruit. You will notice that ladyfingers are very dry and crisp. The fruit juices are going to combine and soak into the biscuits as your trifle develops its flavor in the fridge overnight.

My brother and I always used to fight over who got the most "bottom". As the juices soak through the biscuits the bottom of the trifle becomes, in our opinion, the most flavorful part of the trifle and certainly worth fighting for.

Ingredients

A trifle is a layered dessert of ladyfingers or cake and soft fruits. I'm telling you how we make it in our family and I certainly hope you will try it as I describe at least once. That being said there are no rules as to the fruit mixture you use. Strawberries are popular, in fact any berry works well. As does kiwi, pineapple, banana, peach, mango and papaya. Stick with soft fruits - apples for example don't work and neither does citrus.

My Way

Since trifle is often served at special occasions tradition probably plays a big part in the choice of ingredients. This is how we make it because this is how we have always made it.

Along with the ladyfingers you will need a package of frozen raspberries (thawed) and a can of fruit cocktail. Drain the juice from both into a large measuring cup.

Place a layer of ladyfingers in the bottom of your trifle bowl and spread them with some of the raspberries. Go ahead and break the biscuits to fill in the bottom, as you need to - but don't crush them.

If you are using a deep straight-sided trifle bowl you can line the straight sides with perpendicular ladyfingers for an attractive presentation.

Add some of the mixed fruit to the layer keeping in mind that you will be making 3, 4 or more layers.

Also, on each layer, add a handful of walnut pieces. Large pieces are better and not too many. You want people to discover the walnuts as a treat, not get a mouthful of them. I don't recommend substituting any other nut. Walnuts are soft and have the right mouth feel with this dessert. A crunch would not taste right.

Keep adding layers until you are about 3 inches from the top of the bowl.

BOOZE OR NOT

Now you have to make a choice. Mother's "traditional" trifle has sherry in it. If you choose to add sherry, use Harvey's Bristol Cream, which is a sweet sherry. Dry sherry does not go well with the sweet fruit juices.

Personally I like sherry but I prefer it in a glass, so I usually add a little lemon juice instead. You can squeeze your own or use the ready-squeezed lemon juice from the supermarket.

Whichever you choose, add the sherry or the lemon juice (not both) to the juice in the measuring cup. You can use an ounce or two of sherry, or a tablespoon of lemon juice, but it should be to taste. So, perhaps, start with a little less and taste the juice after each addition until it tastes right to you. You should have about a cup of liquid. If not, add another package of raspberries or a can of fruit cocktail.

[You read this book all the way through before starting your first trifle - right?]

The actual amount of liquid will take some trial and error. You will need more for sponge cake than for ladyfingers and obviously the bigger bowl you use the more of everything you will need.

Taste the juice mixture and adjust for the right balance between fruit and tart.

Gently pour the juice all over the top layer of the trifle, trying to cover it evenly.

It may not look like it now but the juice will soak through all the layers and add its flavor to the ladyfingers. It may take you a couple of tries to get the amount of liquid just right but avoid the temptation to add too much at first. You want the biscuits on the bottom to be moist but not swimming in juice.

Traditional Additions

In the interest of historical accuracy, I should point out that I have omitted six-penny pieces as one of the ingredients. Traditionally, for kids' birthdays, Mother would include a few coins (she boiled them first) for them to discover. I don't recommend you try this unless you have a really good dental plan.

The same is true for ball bearings. No, not literally that's just what I called the tiny silver ball decorations that mother put on top. The traditional name for this confection is nonpareils. Those things were real teeth chippers if you bit them the wrong way.

Toppings

Birds Custard

The next step is custard. Birds Custard to be specific. This custard powder is available in every grocery store in England, most supermarkets in Canada and Australia but, sadly, only in a few imported food sections or specialty food stores in the USA. Amazon has it listed and there is lots of information online about it. If you don't know what Birds Custard is, or have never heard of it, I encourage you to Google it.

I have seen American trifle recipes that use instant pudding for the topping but this is not a viable substitute. Make the effort to get Birds Custard if you can. You will see two sets of directions on the can - one for a sauce and one for a dessert. You want the dessert instructions, as this will make a thicker custard. You need enough to make about a one-inch layer on top of your trifle. You'll have to make an educated guess depending on the size of the bowl you're using.

Pour the prepared custard gently into the bowl and try to create uniform coverage. Now, cover the bowl with plastic wrap and leave it in the fridge until you are ready to serve it.

As custard cools it forms a skin that many people consider a treat. I don't, and so make sure the plastic wrap is in contact with the custard as it cools. This stops the air from getting at it and forming the skin.

Real Whipped Cream

Just before you bring the trifle to the table, add a layer of whipped cream - not Cool Whip or the whipped cream in a spray can - real whipped cream. If you've never made real whipped cream before, it's pretty easy.

MAKING REAL WHIPPED CREAM

Purchase Heavy Whipping Cream from the grocery store. Chill the bowl you'll be using to whip the cream in, particularly if you're in a warm climate. Also chill the beater(s) you are going to use. You can use a hand whisk to whip the cream, but I find it a lot easier to use an electric mixer - many of them come with whisk attachments, or a stick-type electric mixer, which also usually comes with a whisk attachment.

Pour some of the cream into the chilled bowl. How much will be dependent on the size of the bowl. Don't forget that whipped cream is going to have way more volume, so you need to allow for that.

Slowly increase the speed on your electric mixer. If you start at too high a speed you're going to have cream flying everywhere! For the same reason make sure you have sufficient cream in your bowl to cover at least half your beater. It's best to use a small, deep bowl, one with high sides, for whipping cream.

As you're mixing add a little bit of sugar - ¼ cup (50g) should be plenty - and a teaspoon (5mL) of vanilla or almond extract.

Keep beating the whipping cream until it reaches the consistency of - well - whipped cream!

Carefully top your trifle with large dollops of the freshly made whipped cream. Then, drop a few maraschino cherries on top for decoration.

And, there you have it, your very own, authentic English trifle.

It takes a while for the fruit juice to make it to the bottom of the bowl and soften all the biscuits so make your trifle one or two days before you plan to serve it.

SUBSTITUTE CUSTARD

If you can't find Birds Custard in your supermarket and you don't want to order it online you can make it yourself from regular ingredients. Birds Custard is mostly cornstarch and you can even substitute flour if you wish. If you are going to use the substitute my suggestion would be to make some first and try it. Don't risk all the ingredients in your trifle if you need to practice with your custard recipe.

INGREDIENTS

   ½ cup (60g) cornstarch (or plain flour)
   ¼ cup (50g) white or soft brown sugar for better color
   ½ teaspoon (2.5 mL) vanilla essence (to taste)
   4 cups (950 mL) cold milk

OPTIONAL

1 large egg
6 - 8 drops of yellow food coloring

Alfred Bird invented Birds Custard because his wife was allergic to eggs, which was the traditional way of thickening custard. If you use flour you must add the egg to get the mixture to thicken properly. Otherwise it is optional.

Without food colouring your custard will look pasty white and unappetizing. Birds is the color of ripe bananas but that in no way affects the taste.

METHOD

Beat egg, sugar and vanilla essence together. Add about ½ cup (120mL) of the milk, stirring until the sugar is dissolved. Then gradually add the cornstarch to the remaining milk while stirring constantly. You want to avoid lumps.

Put both mixtures in a large heavy bottom saucepan and slowly heat them, stirring constantly. As it gets hot it will thicken. It will thicken very quickly as the mixture gets hot so it is important that you stir it to avoid lumps.

It is very easy to burn the mixture on the bottom of the saucepan so don't try to hurry the process by turning up the heat too much.

When it has the consistency of honey remove from heat and pour over your trifle.

Trifle Recap

Ingredients

Ladyfingers - 3 or 4 packages
Frozen raspberries (or other soft fruit such a strawberries) - 1 to 2 packages
Fruit cocktail - 1 to 2 cans
Juice reserved from raspberries and fruit cocktail
Walnut pieces
Sherry or lemon juice
Whipped cream
A few maraschino cherries

Method

Create layers of ladyfingers, raspberries, fruit cocktail and a few walnut pieces until you're about 3 inches (7.5 cm) from the top of the trifle bowl.

Mix the sherry (or lemon juice) with the reserved juice and evenly pour over the ladyfingers and fruit layers.

Make enough Birds custard (or substitute) to create an approximately one-inch layer (2.5 cm) on the top of your trifle.

Cover the trifle with plastic wrap and refrigerate until just before serving.

Just before serving, make fresh whipped cream and dollop it evenly over the top of the trifle, add a few maraschino cherries for decoration and serve.

Fools

British Fools

From this section title, you could be forgiven for thinking it might be a Monty Python skit. But, no, a "Fool" is actually a specific British dessert type, and very tasty I might add.

They are mostly made with fresh fruit and fresh cream and are particularly welcome and refreshing as a summer dessert.

I choose to include fools in this book because they date back to approximately the same period in history as the trifle.

The "Foole" desert is first mentioned in 1598, as is the trifle but no one seems to know why a fruit dessert is called a fool.

Originally, the most common fruit used was the gooseberry, although apples, strawberries, raspberries and rhubarb are also, very definitely, "authentic".

Gooseberry Fool

You don't see gooseberries in stores much in North America and that's a pity. They're a wonderful fruit.

I like to grow my own and currently have three bushes that are producing fairly well. Enough, at least, to have a few Gooseberry Fools through the season.

Ingredients

> 1½ cups (250g) ripe gooseberries, washed and stems removed
> 3 tablespoons (40g) granulated sugar
> 2 tablespoons (30 mL) water
> ¾ cup (180 mL) Greek yogurt
> 2 tablespoons (13g) icing sugar
> 1 tsp (5 mL) vanilla extract
> ¾ cup (180 mL) heavy cream (whipping cream)

Method

In a saucepan, place the gooseberries, sugar and water. Over medium heat, cook until the gooseberries start to burst, stirring frequently.

Remove from heat and mash the gooseberries with a potato masher until reduced to a pulp.

Set aside until cool and then refrigerate until cold.

In a medium bowl, combine the yogurt, icing sugar and vanilla and beat until smooth.

Whisk in the heavy cream until the mixture thickens nicely.

Gently fold in the gooseberry pulp and carefully spoon the completed mixture into dessert dishes.

Chill for at least an hour before serving.

> *Hint: Want a little "tang" in your fool? Replace half of the Greek yogurt with sour cream!*

Blackberry Fool

I always loved blackberries as a kid. They would grow wild near where I lived and I'd pick copious amounts.

Blackberries in North America, to my mind anyway, don't seem to have as much taste as those I remember from my boyhood days but it may just be a perception thing.

Ingredients

    3½ cups (500g) blackberries, well washed, divided
    ½ cup (100g) granulated sugar
    Juice of 1 lemon
    2 teaspoons (10 mL) vanilla extract
    1½ cups (350 mL) heavy cream (whipping cream)
    ¾ cup (180 mL) Greek yogurt

Method

In a large saucepan, combine 3 cups (425g) of the blackberries, the sugar, lemon juice and vanilla.

Over medium heat, bring the blackberry mixture to a a boil.

Simmer for 3 to 4 minutes. Remove from heat and cool completely.

In a large bowl, whisk the cream until it forms soft peaks.

Gently fold in the yogurt.

Gently fold in a third of the cooled blackberry mixture.

In chilled dessert dishes, layer the rest of the cooled blackberry mixture with the cream mixture.

Garnish with the reserved fresh blackberries.

Serve immediately or refrigerate for up to two hours.

    Hint: Want a little "tang" in your fool? Replace half of the Greek yogurt with sour cream!

Rhubarb Fool

Rhubarb is an oft overlooked dessert option. I'm not really sure why. I'm a big rhubarb fan. I have several plants growing in my yard and harvest rhubarb stalks regularly.

It may seem a bit tart to some people. However, if that's the case, just add a little extra sugar.

Ingredients

- 1 pound (450g) rhubarb, cleaned and chopped into 1 inch pieces
- ¼ cup (45g) light brown sugar
- 1¼ cups (300 mL) heavy cream (whipping cream)
- ½ cup (120 mL) Greek yogurt
- Small bunch of mint, leaves only (optional)

Method

In a medium saucepan, combine the rhubarb and brown sugar. Cook over medium-low heat until just tender. - DO NOT OVERCOOK - Remove from heat as soon as soft.

Test for sweetness and add more sugar if required.

Drain the rhubarb, reserving the juice.

Allow the rhubarb to cool and then refrigerate until cold.

In a medium bowl, whip the cream until it forms soft peaks and then stir in the yogurt.

Gently fold in the chilled rhubarb and carefully spoon the completed mixture into dessert dishes.

Chill for at least an hour before serving.

When serving, top with the reserved rhubarb juice and mint leaves, if desired.

Note: Do not eat rhubarb leaves! They contain an ingredient that will make you very sick.

Strawberry Fool

There's nothing like fresh strawberries in season. This no-cook dessert takes advantage of their natural sweetness and appealing color.

Ingredients

> 2 cups (400g) strawberries, washed, hulled and chopped (Note: reserve one or two strawberries to be sliced for garnish)
> ½ cup (100g) granulated sugar, divided
> 1 cup (240 mL) heavy cream (whipping cream)
> 1 teaspoon (5 mL) vanilla extract

Method

Combine the chopped strawberries with ¼ cup (50g) sugar. Toss and allow to sit for 10 to 15 minutes, stirring occasionally, until juice forms.

Pour off the juice into a blender, combine with half of the chopped strawberries and puree.

Combine the puree with the other half of the chopped strawberries.

Whisk the cream with the remaining sugar and vanilla until cream has thickened and peaks begin to form.

Gently fold the berries into the mixture and carefully spoon the completed fool into dessert dishes.

Garnish with strawberry slices and serve immediately or refrigerate for up to two hours.

> *Hint: There is a huge difference in taste between locally grown strawberries, in season, and the ones you get off season that are picked green and trucked for thousands of miles.*
>
> *Do your taste buds a favour and only make your fools in season from local strawberries.*

Strawberry Rhubarb Fool

Even those who say they're not fans of rhubarb often enjoy the strawberry-rhubarb taste combination - particularly in a pie!

This Fool recipe takes advantage of this blend of flavors to create a lighter dessert that's still packed with taste.

> *Pop quiz - how many of you have accidentally said rawberry-strhubarb? Come on. It can't just be me!*

Ingredients

½ pound (225g) rhubarb, cleaned and chopped into 1 inch pieces
1 cup (200g) strawberries, washed, hulled and chopped (Note: reserve one or two strawberries to be sliced for garnish)
¼ cup (45g) light brown sugar
1¼ cups (300 mL) heavy cream (whipping cream)
½ cup (120 mL) Greek yogurt
Small bunch of mint, leaves only (optional)

Method

In a medium saucepan, combine the rhubarb, strawberries and brown sugar.

Cook over medium-low heat until the rhubarb is just tender.

Test mixture for sweetness and add more sugar if required.

Drain the rhubarb-strawberry mixture and reserve the juice.

Allow the mixture to cool and then refrigerate until cold.

In a medium bowl, whip the cream until it forms soft peaks and then stir in the yogurt.

Gently fold in the chilled rhubarb-strawberry mixture and carefully spoon the completed mixture into dessert dishes.

Chill for at least an hour before serving.

When serving, top with the reserved juice, strawberry slices and mint leaves, if desired.

Raspberry Fool

This Raspberry Fool (no-cook) recipe can be made with or without a raspberry liqueur (such as Chambord), your choice.

Either way, it's a great way to make a dessert with seasonable, fresh raspberries.

Raspberries not in season? Check the bottom of the recipe for a hack you can use when you can't get fresh raspberries.

Ingredients

3 cups (375g) raspberries, reserve a few for garnish
1/4 cup (50g) granulated sugar
3 tablespoons (45 mL) raspberry liqueur, such as Chambord (or substitute water)
2 cups (475 mL) heavy cream
1/2 cup (50g) powdered (confectioner's) sugar
Fresh Mint Sprigs, For Garnish (optional)

Method

In a medium bowl, combine the raspberries (reserving a few for garnish), granulated sugar and liqueur (or water).

Stir well and let it sit for 10 to 15 minutes.

In a larger bowl, whip the cream with the powdered sugar until it forms soft peaks.

Mash the raspberries with a fork until all the liquid and fruit are mashed together.

Spoon half of the fruit mixture into the whipped cream and gently fold once or twice being careful not to over mix.

Add the remaining fruit mixture and fold once or twice.

Carefully spoon the completed mixture into chilled dessert glasses, garnish with whole raspberries and mint sprigs, if desired.

Serve immediately.

> *Note: Of course you always have the option of substituting frozen raspberries but they tend to be full of liquid. Drain well before using. You can use this liquid to make a raspberry tea.*

BONUS! - Raspberry Hack

Recipe hack for when fresh or frozen raspberries aren't available.

INGREDIENTS

    1 cup (325g) raspberry jam
    3 tablespoons (45 mL) raspberry liqueur, such as Chambord (or substitute water)
    2 cups (475 mL) heavy cream
    ½ cup (50g) powdered (confectioner's) sugar
    Fresh Mint Sprigs, For Garnish (optional)

In a small bowl, combine the raspberry jam and liqueur (or water). Mix well.

In a larger bowl, whip the cream with the powdered sugar until it forms soft peaks.

Spoon half of the jam mixture into the whipped cream and gently fold once or twice being careful not to over mix.

Add the remaining jam mixture and fold once or twice.

Carefully spoon the completed mixture into chilled dessert glasses and garnish with mint sprigs, if desired.

Serve immediately.

Mango Fool

Definitely not Authentic English but we have a huge Mango tree in our garden and have difficulty using all the fruit.

So how about a tropical fool? The taste of a fresh, ripe mango lends itself perfectly to a delightfully light and creamy fool.

This is also a no-cook recipe, so no need to heat up the kitchen on a warm summer day.

Ingredients

>1 medium ripe mango, peeled, pitted and chopped, reserving a few slices for garnish
>3 tablespoons (38g) granulated sugar
>2 teaspoons (10 mL) freshly squeezed lime juice (about 1/2 lime)
>1 cup (240 mL) heavy cream (whipping cream)
>½ teaspoon (2.5 mL) vanilla extract

Method

In a blender, combine the chopped mango, 2 tablespoons (25g) of sugar and the lime juice. Blend until smooth.

In a large bowl whisk the heavy cream with the remaining tablespoon sugar and the vanilla, until soft peak form.

Set aside 1/2 cup (120 mL) of the whipped cream for garnish.

Gently fold the mango puree into the remaining whipped cream until combined. Carefully spoon the mango mixture into chilled dessert dishes.

Garnish with the reserved whipped cream and mango slices.

Serve immediately or refrigerate for up to two hours.

BEEF STEW

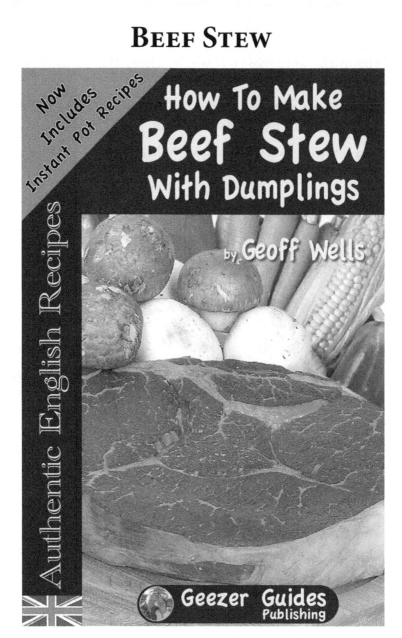

How to Make a Perfect Stew Every Time

Beef - Chicken - Lamb - Vegetable - Ham - Turkey

A stew, in the most basic terms, is water flavored with meat and vegetables. But, if you just throw everything into a pot and boil it, you're not likely to get the results you were hoping for.

A good, hearty, flavorful stew is simple to make but very few people, in my experience, seem to be able to get it right.

There are a few rules you need to learn that apply to pretty much any boiled dinner.

Rule #1 Don't Boil

Simmer is good, boil is bad. To simmer means that small bubbles just break the surface. When that happens, then you have the temperature just right. Don't try to rely on setting your stove at some particular mark – you need to use your eyes - the setting will need to be adjusted depending on the weather, what you are cooking and what you are cooking it in.

Rule #2 Don't Use Too Much Water

You use water to dilute so many things, doesn't it make sense that if you add a lot of water to your stew you will dilute the flavor. Of course, you should try to start with a stock rather than water, but we'll get to that later.

Rule #3 Make Your Stew at Least a Day Before You Plan to Serve It

You want to give your stew's flavor the opportunity to develop. You also want the stew to cool so you can remove any fat from the surface. This is particularly important when you are making ham, chicken or turkey stew, which can be especially greasy.

Rule #4 Use Premium Ingredients

I suppose it's tempting to try to get rid of all the leftovers in the fridge by making a stew out of them. But that won't make a stew you will be proud of. A piece of stringy celery, a lump of fat or meat you can't chew can spoil even the best tasting dinner.

Rule #5 Taste It Before You Serve It

Don't be as surprised as everyone else if your stew doesn't taste right. There are ways to fix most disasters. So, before you throw it out and call for take-out, read on.

Stock

As I mentioned above, you should always start your stew with stock if at all possible. For most of your stews the meat and vegetables you use won't provide enough flavor to the water on their own.

If you plan to make a stew in a day or two, save any of the water you use to boil potatoes, carrots, cabbage, etc. and put it in the fridge to use as stock.

Any time you boil your vegetables, a lot of the goodness and flavor ends up in the water that you throw away. Steaming is much better but then you don't have much liquid left for stock.

Another option is to buy a can or tetra pack of broth. You can get beef, chicken and vegetable broth at most grocery stores. This will give your stew an excellent start.

There are a few cases when you will want to start by boiling some bones - ham, chicken or turkey stew for example. It's a good idea to make stock from any kind of bones, however, today we don't seem to see beef bones. When I was younger, my mother would get soup bones from our local butcher but it's not something you see in the supermarkets today.

I should qualify that last statement that I'm talking about the USA. England still has real butcher shops and many Canadian supermarkets still have butchers on staff that can supply bones and even kidney or suet if you ask. I don't know, but I imagine Australia and New Zealand are much the same.

In other words, if you're reading this in the USA, you're most likely going to have to use a can of broth.

I got a little sidetracked with the bones. I was talking about ham and poultry.

Ham shoulders usually have a large bone in the middle that you end up throwing away. Don't. Put the bone in a heavy pot, big enough to hold it, cover it with water and simmer it for an hour or two.

Remove the bone and give it to your (or your neighbor's) dog. Put the pot in the fridge (after it has cooled). When it is well chilled, remove the fat that has hardened on the top of the jelly. Yes, I said jelly. Don't worry, it will liquify as soon as you warm it up.

Have you ever weighed your turkey leftovers? I'm not talking about the half dozen plastic wrapped packages in the freezer you are saving for sandwiches. I'm talking about the skin, bones and giblets you throw in the garbage when you cook a whole turkey.

You might be surprised that it is almost 50% of the weight of your original turkey. But don't throw it all out. You can use it to make the most marvelous stock for your stews and soups.

Do the same as you did with the ham bone. Put everything in a big, heavy pot - the skin, bones, giblets, leftover stuffing, any jelly off the carving plate - all of it. Cover with water and simmer for a couple of hours. Let it cool then strain the resulting stock into a bowl.

First, use a slotted spoon to lift out the largest pieces of bone, then pour what's left through a sieve to catch all the small bones and pieces of turkey that have now been cooked to death.

Grease

Put the strained liquid in the fridge to chill so that you can remove any fat. The chilled fat will float to the top and harden, making it easy to remove.

I'm not telling you to remove the fat for health reasons - although that is a very good reason - you just don't want your stew to have a greasy taste.

It's always a good idea to put a handful of rice in any stew that is potentially greasy - particularly chicken and turkey.

Split Peas

Split peas go very well with ham and will add lots of flavor and body to your soup or stew. The only problem is that they take a long time to cook. If you put them in with the other ingredients, they will still be like little bullets when your carrots are just right. If you cook them long enough so that they soften then your potato chunks will have disappeared into the liquid.

The solution, of course, is to make them part of the stock and cook them long enough to be incorporated into the stock. You can hurry the process along a bit by using a blender to smooth out your stock.

Yellow Split Peas Pudding

OK, this has nothing to do with making stews, so consider it a bonus.

You can use split peas to make an interesting substitute for your usual rice or potatoes. All you do is boil them long enough to absorb all the water you are cooking them in.

Start out with, say, 1 cup (240 mL) of yellow split peas to 2 cups (480 mL) of water. Use a saucepan with a heavy bottom and keep simmering until all the water is absorbed. If the peas still aren't soft just add a little more water and keep cooking. You should end up with a smooth paste much like the consistency of mashed potatoes.

Recipes

Up until now I haven't mentioned any recipes and I only bring it up because you may be wondering where they are. You will find my grandmother's beef stew recipe at the end but, for the most part, making soups and stews is more about a process and most of the time you'll just wing it.

Certainly there are specialty soups and stews, like gazpacho, mulligatawny and beef bourguignon, where you need a recipe to follow the first time, but for everyday meals you will learn what works together and make your standard dishes much the same each time.

Don't get hung up on recipes. This booklet is about method, once you have that mastered you will use recipes as suggestions and springboards to inspiration.

Vegetables

You can put almost any vegetable you like into your stew and the resulting flavor will change either slightly or significantly - depending on how strong a flavor the vegetable has and how much you use.

As a minimum, I always like to start with carrots and onions. Next would be celery, potatoes and cabbage.

I like peppers in a salad but in a stew they can take over the flavor if you use too much. The same is true for celery root.

Zucchini is okay but does not add much flavor and goes mushy if cooked too long. It's best to add any soft vegetables like this during the last 10 minutes before the stew is done.

If you are one of those people who will only eat the very top of broccoli, then a stew is a great way to use the stalks you would otherwise throw away. Just keep the stalks in a baggie in the freezer until you need them. Don't go crazy with this veggie, though. Try not to use any more than a two-inch thick stalk, but up to a half-inch thick piece of stalk is fine. Leave it in bite size pieces or chop it up either way it makes a great addition to your stew.

You see what I mean about winging it. Use quality ingredients and some common sense. Put in what you like and it will be fine.

Spices

With a few exceptions, I don't add many spices. My wife likes to add a couple of bay leaves (particularly to a ham stew) but, personally, I don't think they make much difference.

I usually add a couple of shakes of Worcestershire sauce and a bouillon cube, which we'll talk about in a minute.

The exception is turkey stew, which, in my opinion, is greatly improved with sage. If you stuff your turkey with a sage and onion stuffing, and some of the leftover stuffing makes it into the stock, then you will get some of the flavor. But, be sure to taste it to see if you need to add some.

Bouillon

A watery stew may still be full of goodness but it doesn't taste very good. Kick your taste up a notch or two by adding a bouillon cube or liquid towards the end of the cooking process.

My favorites, in order, are Bovril™, OXO™ and Knorr™. I think you can get them in most grocery stores in the Western world although in the USA you may have to look in the imported foods section.

You can also get store brands and bouillon cubes from the dollar store, but watch out for the salt content. Some of these imitations are so salty they can ruin your meal.

Salt

I often add a teaspoonful (5 mL) or two to a 3 quart (2.85 L) saucepan of stew. It really helps to bring out the flavor - but taste it before and after. Add just a little at a time. You can always add more salt, if needed, but you can't take it out.

And, watch out for the cheap bouillon cubes. Try spooning out some of your stew into a measuring cup and dissolving your cube in that before adding it to the pot. This way, if it is super-salty, you can toss it in the garbage without ruining all your hard work.

The Process

OK, I think you have enough background, it's time to put it all together and make a stew.

If you are making a red meat stew from scratch you start with the meat but I'm including my "Perfect Every Time Beef Stew Recipe" at the end so for now we'll cover stews from leftovers.

Since the ham, chicken or turkey is already cooked, it gets added right at the end because all you want to do is warm it up.

We've already talked about how important the stock is, but if you don't have any you can use water and some extra bouillon.

Prepare Your Vegetables

At a minimum, you'll need a medium to large yellow onion and 3 or 4 carrots. If you can find carrots that still have their green tops, that's best, otherwise you will have to settle for the ones in the poly bag. Just make sure they are reasonably fresh and break with a snap. If you cut the carrots in wheels their flavor tends to get lost. I prefer 1 to 2 inch (2.5 to 5 cm) pieces so that when you eat them you get the full carrot taste. The same goes for the onions, if you finely chop them you will flavor the stew water but you won't get the same taste experience that you do from a decent bite-size piece.

You might want to consider keeping all your vegetables to bite-size so that each mouthful has its own distinct taste.

Bring your stock to a simmer and add the vegetables that take the longest to cook. Onion, carrots and celery should be first in the pot.

By adding the vegetables to the stock, the stock will no longer be simmering, so adjust the heat to achieve a nice simmer and put the lid on the pot. Covering the pot will raise the temperature so you will have to turn the heat down to avoid boiling it and to maintain a slow simmer.

Note: Stew should never be boiled.

After a few minutes add potato, cabbage, broccoli, etc. and continue to simmer.

Finally, add any watery vegetables like yams and zucchini.

When you can easily stick a fork in a piece of carrot, the stew is done. Time to taste it and adjust the flavors.

Add teaspoons of Bovril™ or OXO™ cubes one at a time, tasting in between, until it is right. If you add more than 2 or 3 you probably started with too much water.

Thickening

Consistency is important to a successful stew. If you used a split pea stock your liquid will be thicker than water but may still benefit from thickening.

In days gone by, cooks (and some chefs today) used a flour roux to thicken stews. It works but can be tricky to use and often leads to clumps of raw flour in your liquid.

Cornstarch is much easier to use and the results are fairly consistent. The famous Escoffier Cookbook recommends it over a roux, so that is good enough for me.

Put a couple of teaspoons of cornstarch in a measuring cup and carefully add just enough cold water to make a liquid. Be careful not to add too much water. As you stir the mixture it can seem almost solid and then the next drop of water will be all you need.

Turn up the heat under your pot slightly. Stir your stew and gradually add the cornstarch mixture.

You should see the consistency change. Stop adding the cornstarch as you approach the thickness you are aiming for.

LEFTOVER STEW

What is leftover stew, you ask?

It's a way to use up what ever is left over from the Sunday roast.

Basically you make a vegetable stew as I just described then, as a last step, you add the leftover meat and turn off the heat.

Just be conscious of what you're adding to your stew. The quality of the meat should not be any less than what you served as the Sunday roast. Don't ruin your hard work by using scraps that should be given to the dog. Trim off the fat and gristle. If it's tough, putting it in the stew won't improve it.

> *Growing up, Monday was always laundry day, which meant leftovers for dinner. Without an automatic washer and only a clothes line to dry the clothes and bedding laundry was very hard work and took all day.*
>
> *Yes, I'm that old!*

A Word About Dumplings

I love dumplings but an ever-increasing waistline has forced me to forgo this pleasure. They are easy to make and are a tasty addition to your stews. You add them to your stew just before you serve so don't make them and put them in the fridge overnight.

You can use flour and baking powder but I get best results by using Bisquick™. Again I believe this name brand product is available from most grocery stores in the Western world.

There is a dumpling recipe on the box but the basic idea is to mix powder and milk, form rough balls of dough and drop them in the simmering stew for 15 to 20 minutes. Keep the pot covered because the dumplings float and you want them cooked on the top and bottom.

Don't make the mixture too wet - use about ¾ cup (115g) of Bisquick to ⅓ cup (80mL) of milk. You can add a beaten egg and a little butter or margarine but it is not necessary. One nice touch is to include some fresh chopped parsley or cilantro.

Suet Dumplings

If you want the full authentic experience then you need to make suet dumplings. If you live in the US you might have some difficulty getting suet from your local supermarket but it is available online. Check our website for updated links to all kinds of British products. (https://ebooks.geezerguides.com/products-from-our-books/)

Ingredients

½ cup (60g) flour
¼ cup (50g) shredded suet
¾ teaspoon (4 mL) baking powder
⅛ teaspoon (0.6 mL) salt
5 tablespoons (75 mL) cold water, approximately

Method

Put the flour, suet, baking powder and salt in a small bowl and mix well. Add just enough cold water to make the dough pliable but not sticky.

If it's too sticky add a little more flour.

Put a little flour on your hands and divide the dough into 8 pieces then roll them into balls.

About 20 minutes before your stew is done, drop the balls into the simmering liquid. Keep covered and cook gently for at least 20 minutes.

Servings: 4

Suggestions

You can add some interest by experimenting with various herbs added to your dough. Check out the Atora website (http://www.atora.co.uk) for more dumpling recipes.

When It All Goes Pear-Shaped

If you have used quality ingredients and followed my recommendations, there is not much that could go wrong. I can see just a few possibilities - too thick, too thin, too salty, or no taste.

Too Thick

If it's too thick then you've added too much cornstarch. Maybe you added the mixture when your stew was not quite hot enough and didn't realize you had added too much until the stew reached the right temperature and solidified.

No problem. Just stir in more liquid. Don't use water if you can avoid it because you will dilute the flavor. Use broth if you have it or make up some bouillon in a measuring cup and add that.

Too Thin

If it's too thin just mix up some additional cornstarch and slowly add it to the simmering liquid. Your stew must be almost boiling for the cornstarch to work. It's a chemical process and that's what it takes to activate the cornstarch molecules.

No Taste

If you used a good stock and quality bouillon, then taste should not be a problem. Just add more broth and bouillon.

If all else fails, put everything in a blender and make it into a creamy soup.

No, I'm not patronizing - I've done it. Sometimes that's just how you learn.

Too Salty

Too salty is tricky. Adding rice and potatoes will help to absorb the salt but the only way to dilute the taste, if it can't be rescued with rice or potatoes, is to make a second stew with absolutely no salt and mix the two together.

Best Beef Stew Ever

I am about to share a family recipe that is over one hundred years old. I hope that you will try it exactly as I present it, at least once. If not, you will be missing one of your life's most amazing taste experiences.

Quite a build-up but for many years after I left home I jokingly accused my mother of not sharing the magic ingredients as I was unable to reproduce the flavor I had grown up with.

Turns out it is not so much the ingredients as the process, which is what I have tried to stress in this booklet.

The Beef

There's an old saying about not making a silk purse out of a sow's ear. The same principle applies here. Your finished stew will only be as good as your ingredients and your major ingredient is the beef.

You can generally find shrink-wrapped trays of "stewing beef" in your local supermarket - avoid them. Take a look at some of the inexpensive roasts. Blade or top sirloin roasts are often cheaper per pound than "stewing beef" and will make a much better stew. Get something around 3 - 4 pounds (1.4 - 1.8 Kg). This will make 4 - 6 meals, more if you don't eat much.

Cut the roast into cubes about ¾ - 1 inch (3 cm) on each side. Remember, they will shrink quite a bit when cooked. Make sure you remove any fat, gristle, etc. and watch out for string. Butchers love to tie roasts up in string and it's not very tasty.

Kidney

The Brits said OK, the American said Yuck, Canadians and Australians are probably divided.

Americans can use the excuse that kidney is almost impossible to find in any supermarket. You will need to go to one of the premium chains, like AJ's, and order it specially.

If you're not willing to try it, you are really missing out. If there is a secret ingredient in this recipe - this is it.

One beef kidney is enough to make 5 or 6 stews.

You don't have to eat it but you do need it to flavor the rich gravy. My wife is Canadian and loves the flavor but even after more than a quarter century together she still won't eat any kidney.

Cut the kidney into 5 or 6 pieces and individually wrap and freeze what you don't need. Cut the piece you will use into smaller pieces and remove the strip of fat in the middle.

If you don't plan to eat it, you can leave it in larger chunks, which will make it easier to identify and remove.

Sear the Meat

Dust a small amount of white flour on the cutting board and roll the meat and kidney pieces in it until they are well covered.

Put a heavy bottomed saucepan, big enough to hold everything that's going into your stew on medium heat. Add the beef and kidney to the empty saucepan and toss the meat around until it is well seared.

Add Water

If you have any vegetable stock you can use it but, in this case, because the flavors are so intense, it is okay to use plain water - but not too much. Just cover the meat and not a drop more.

Both the meat and the vegetables have water content, which they lose during cooking. The meat will shrink and you will end up with more liquid than you thought.

Bring the water to a simmer, but don't let it reach a rolling boil.

Add Vegetables

All you are going to add is carrots and onions. One large onion, sliced, but not chopped and up to half a dozen carrots cut in bite-size pieces. Carrots vary a lot in size, so use your own judgment.

Bovril™

Add a tablespoon (15 mL) of Bovril™ or dissolve 2 OXO™ beef cubes in a measuring cup with hot water. Stir into the mixture.

Cook Slowly

Cover and cook slowly for about an hour. Try to keep it at a slow, steady simmer and let the carrots tell you when it is done. If your fork goes in easily, it is done.

Taste It

Taste it to see if you need more salt or Bovril™.

You can remove the kidney now, if you are not going to eat it. Your dog or cat will just love it.

THICKEN IT

All that is left now is to thicken the stew with cornstarch. This is something that is so easy to do but difficult to write about. All I can think of is that it should be about the consistency of motor oil. Not a very appetizing analogy but at least you get the idea. Growing up, my daughter used to call it chocolate gravy.

LET THE FLAVORS MATURE

Pop the cooled saucepan into the fridge overnight. Next day, heat the stew and add dumplings if you wish. Serve with mashed potatoes and fresh peas.

STEAK AND KIDNEY PIE

If you really want a treat, you can combine this stew recipe with my wife Vicky's pastry recipe for a steak and kidney pie that will have your guests begging for more.

"[How To Make Perfect Pastry Every Time](#)" **by Vicky Wells**

Recipe Recap

Simmer - Don't Boil

Boiling your stew can ruin it. Keep it at a low, steady simmer. A simmer means that tiny bubbles just barely break the surface of the liquid.

Quality Ingredients

Always start with quality ingredients - meat and vegetables.

Stock

If at all possible, use stock, not plain water as your base. Stock can be as simple as keeping the water that you cooked vegetables in. Or, you can create your own stock by boiling beef bones, ham bones, chicken or turkey carcasses. See the instructions for that in this book under Stock.

Vegetables

Use quality vegetables. At the very least, use carrots and onions. Don't cut your veggies too small. Slice the onions and leave the carrots in chunks about 1½ inches (4 cm) to 2 inches (5 cm) long. Carrots are a good way to determine when your stew is done. When you can easily stick a fork in the carrots, the stew is done. Always put the vegetables that need more cooking time (onions, carrots, celery) in the simmering stock first.

Preparing a Stew with Pre-Cooked Meat

This kind of preparation works well with leftover ham, turkey or chicken. Quality is important so only use cooked meats that you would serve to guests, not the scraps that you would otherwise give to the dog or throw out.

Prepare the stock, add the veggies, thicken and THEN add the pre-cooked meat.

Beef Stew - Or Other Red Meats

The best recipe is right here in this booklet. Follow the instructions, including adding the kidney - really.

Let the Flavors Mature

For any stew you make, let it rest in the fridge overnight so the flavors have a chance to blend and mature. Trust me on this one.

Now that you've read everything, it's time to make your own stew. Follow the instructions, use quality ingredients and you'll do just fine. And remember, simmer - don't boil.

Instant Pot - Best Beef Stew Ever

The Instant Pot excels at stew and with this recipe you will be sure to make the best beef stew you have ever tasted.

Ingredients

3 pounds (1.5 Kg) blade or top sirloin roast, cut into ¾ - 1 inch (2 - 2.5 cm) cubes
1 large onion, cut in bite size pieces
3 - 4 large carrots, cut into 1 inch (2.5 cm) pieces
1 tablespoon (15 mL) Bovril™
1 teaspoon (5 mL) salt, or to taste
Stock to cover
3 ounces (85g) beef kidney, cut into 6 pieces (optional but recommended)
2 teaspoons (10 mL) cornstarch (or sufficient)

Method

1. Dust the beef and kidney with unbleached all purpose flour.
2. Press the Sauté key on the Instant Pot and add the beef and kidney to the stainless steel inner pot, stirring vigorously to prevent the meat from sticking.
3. When the meat is seared, pour in just enough stock to cover the meat.
4. Add the carrots, onions, Bovril™ and salt.
5. Close the lid and turn the vent to Sealing
6. Click the Meat/Stew button add set the time to 30 minutes.
7. When the time is up Quick release to vent the steam
8. Mix the cornstarch with just enough water to make it liquid and stir it into the stew. If the stew doesn't thicken you may have to turn on Sauté for a few minutes to bring to simmer while stirring.
9. You can serve it right away but the flavours will mature if you leave it until tomorrow.

Liver & Onions

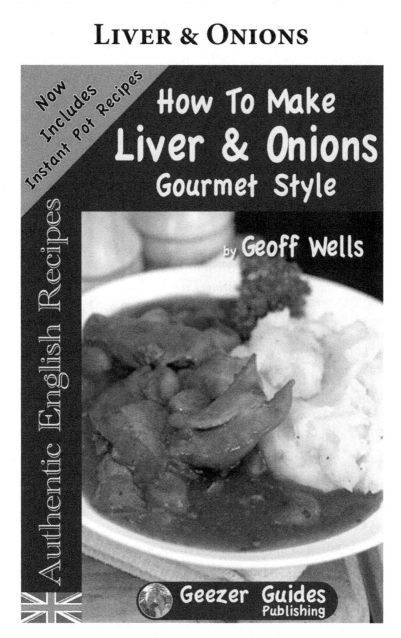

GOURMET STYLE LIVER AND ONIONS DINNER

All chefs have their signature dish - the one they consider to be their best - the recipe that defines their culinary skill. I'm not a chef but this would be my signature dish if I was.

Liver and onions may seem like a strange choice for this exalted position but you haven't tasted it yet. My wife hated liver when we first met - but I will let her tell the story :

"That's right, I didn't just dislike liver, I HATED it! I had never been able to cook liver so that I liked the results and, even as a kid, when my Mom would cook liver I couldn't even choke it down.

So, when Geoff and I were first dating, when he announced that he was going to cook dinner for me I was thrilled. Then he told me it would be liver and onions. Oh, no! As we had just started dating I resigned myself to having to not only choke it down, but to try very hard to look like I liked it. This wasn't going to be easy.

If my body language gave away my trepidation, then either Geoff didn't notice or he chose to ignore it.

On the fateful evening I sat down at the table, trying to be as positive and cheerful as possible. However, if I left most of it on my plate, or worse still, spit it out, would there be another date? We were about to find out.

Initially I cut myself a very small piece of the liver figuring I could at least swallow a small bit without gagging.

But, wait a sec, can this actually be liver? It tasted good! Very good! I had never had a liver dinner prepared in this way.

I didn't have to fake it at all. I truly enjoyed the meal and ended up cleaning my plate.

And, yes, there were many more dates and we've now been married for almost thirty years and I often ask him to make liver and onions. I also ask him to make it for friends and family, too, who also rave about it."

The secret to this meal is not the recipes - it's the method. A simple listing of ingredients is meaningless and you will not be able to duplicate my results unless you follow my method precisely.

This is a recipe for a meal not just a dish. The liver, onions, bacon, spinach, potatoes and gravy all work together to produce the desired effect.

Liver

Start with the best beef liver you can find. Not calf's liver or chicken liver - beef. A lot of liver sold these days seems to be "fast fry" which is liver cut so thin that it barely stays together. If that is all you can find, it will have to do but what you are looking for is liver slices about $3/8"$ (1 cm) thick. That is just a little thinner than a slice of bread.

Ideally each slice should be free of sinews, fat, etc. Trim off any imperfections and give them to your cat - they'll love it.

Be very particular about cutting out any holes. That may sound silly but the holes are blood vessels and are lined with tough sinew. If you or your guests gets one they may not be able to swallow it.

How much you need will obviously depend on how many you are serving but you should allow, on average, two pieces per person. Each piece being about 3 to 5 inches (7.5 to 12.5 cm) long by 2 to 3 inches (5 to 7.5 cm) wide. I only mention the size so you have some idea how much you need. I'm not suggesting that you have to serve it in those sizes but if you are concerned about presentation then try to keep each piece a uniform size.

You can also cook up some extra because your guests are going to want seconds.

Bacon

You would think I could just specify bacon and everyone would know what I mean but the term bacon means something different depending on where you live.

English Bacon

English bacon is quite meaty with very little fat. It looks like a roughly 2 to 3 inch (5 - 7.5 cm) diameter squashed circle of meat connected to a 4 or 5 inch (10 or 12 cm) tail of meat and fat.

American Bacon

American bacon is just the "tail" section of English bacon. I don't know what the meaty end is sold as. If you know the answer, please let me know.

Canadian Bacon

Here again, there are two types of Canadian bacon - what you buy in Canada and what you buy in the USA. In Canada the meaty end of English bacon is called peameal bacon and is sold by the piece rather than sliced and is covered in cornmeal. In the US "Canadian bacon" is sold in vacuum packed slices without the cornmeal. It is also sometimes called "back bacon". Canadians also eat "regular bacon" which is the same as American bacon.

Which Bacon To Use?

As much as I like English bacon, for this meal the American Bacon is a better choice. This is because we will use the bacon fat to fry the liver. In England you will will just have to add some dripping* or butter to the pan.

Dripping

My mother always saved the fat from the Sunday roast in a basin (bowl). This was then used in cooking or spread on toast. The jelly in the bottom of the dish was a particular delicacy. (Vicky says ugh!)

Spinach

Please don't try to substitute some other green vegetable - it won't produce the same results. The juice from the spinach is an essential ingredient to the gravy.

Baby Spinach

Over the past few years it seems that baby spinach has replaced regular spinach, at least in the stores we go to. This is good because it takes far less preparation. If you have a choice, definitely go for the baby spinach.

Regular Spinach

If you buy regular spinach you will need to inspect each leaf and remove the part of the stalk that is below the leaf. This is because cooking the spinach the way we do the old stalks might not cook down and be "woody". While you are washing it, cut off each stalk before you put the leaf in the saucepan.

Cooking Spinach

Thoroughly wash the spinach because it is often grown in sandy soil and you need to remove any trace of grit. Spinach is mostly water and cooks down more than any other vegetable. You can start with a large saucepan stuffed with leaves and end up with a couple of tablespoonsful to serve.

Never add water to your saucepan full of spinach. What is left on the leaves after washing them is all the water you need.

Baby spinach usually comes in a 10 ounce (285g) bag and you will need about one bag per person - as I said, it cooks down a lot.

After washing transfer it to a large, heavy-bottomed saucepan. Quickly drain the saucepan and cook on a low to medium heat. Be careful not to burn it to the bottom of the saucepan and flip it around a couple of times as it cooks.

Additional Ingredients

Onion

Any ordinary white or yellow onion is fine. I like to use a big one and slice from the top to the root producing rings of onion.

Tip

> *If cutting onions bothers you, leave the root on while you slice it. The chemical that makes your eyes water is in the base of the onion and is released when you cut it. Using fridge cold onions and cutting them under water will also prevent the release of the chemical.*

Whipped Potatoes

I'm always amazed at the comments I get whenever I serve mashed potatoes. I have always whipped them and so think nothing of it but, apparently, this is not normally what people do.

Cut peeled potatoes into 2 inch (5 cm) cubes and boil in salted water until you can stick a fork into them.

How much salt?

To taste, but about a teaspoonful (5 mL). I just pour some into the palm of my hand then dump it in the pot.

When the potatoes are cooked, thoroughly drain them. Then, use a potato masher to break them up as much as possible. Add a little milk or a generous pat of butter. How much is a little? Probably less than ¼ cup (60 mL) but it will vary depending on how many potatoes you cooked.

Use a heavy fork and slowly start to stir in the milk. Increase the speed of your stirring until you are beating the potatoes into a paste. I hold the saucepan in one hand and the fork in the other. Success is all in the wrist action. You don't want mashed potatoes too wet. Try to whip them with as little milk as you can. You can add just the pat of butter and possibly some chopped parsley if you like.

Tip

> *I always hold the saucepan in the sink while I'm doing this in case I get a little carried away and spray mashed potato all over the kitchen.*

In addition to what I have already mentioned, you will need about ½ cup (60 g) of white flour, Bovril™, OXO™ or some other beef bouillon, corn starch and mustard.

Colemans™ Mustard

In the US and Canada mustard means the stuff in the squeeze bottle that you squirt on hamburgers and hot dogs. In England mustard means Colemans dry mustard.

The tastes are completely different. Squeeze bottle stuff is mixed with vinegar and has no kick. You could eat it with a spoon if you were so inclined.

Colemans is hot. You mix a little of the ground mustard seed with just enough water to make a paste and eat it cautiously.

My older brother likes to tell a story about me whining in my highchair wanting to taste the mustard. Apparently he fed me a spoonful of it and I didn't whine for it anymore.

Anyway, liver is traditionally served with hot mustard. It's easy to find in England, Canada and Australia. In the US we've found it in the imported foods section of most big supermarkets.

Putting It All Together

The secret to any successful meal is timing. Make sure everything is ready when it is supposed to be and serve everything hot and fresh.

Step 1 - The Bacon

Start by cooking the bacon in a large frying pan. You will serve about two strips of bacon per person, but go ahead and cook the whole package. You can freeze whatever you don't use or crumble it up for bacon bits.

Over the past few years the water content in bacon has increased significantly and you will need to pour the water off after a couple of minutes of cooking.

When the bacon is as crisp as you like it, remove the strips from the fat and let them drain on a folded paper towel.

Turn on your oven to its lowest setting - around 200 Deg. F (100°C, Gas Mark ½)- and put your dinner plates and the bacon in the oven to keep warm.

Step 2 - The Onion

Put your sliced onion in the bacon fat and cook until the onion is clear. Don't cook onions too fast as they will quickly burn and caramelize.

When they're done, remove them from the pan and place them onto some more paper towel and put them in the oven. Yes, the paper towel is on a plate and, no, it won't catch fire at this low temperature.

Step 3 - The Potatoes

Bring the potatoes to a boil then turn down to simmer until you can but a fork through them. Keep a lid on the pot to better control the heat.

Step 4 - The Spinach

At the same time you start the potatoes, you also start the spinach. But, the spinach you cook on a low to medium heat otherwise you will burn the bottom leaves.

Make sure you have a well-fitting lid because you are more steaming the spinach than boiling it.

Halfway through, check you have the heat high enough. The pot should now only be half as full as it was and you need to stir the still uncooked leaves on the top to the bottom.

Step 5 - The Liver

On a plate or cutting board, spread about ½ cup (60g) of white flour. Drop each piece of liver into the flour and make sure each piece is completely covered with the flour.

Lower each flour-coated piece of liver into the hot bacon fat. You only need enough fat to set the flour. It doesn't have to be "swimming". If you don't have enough, just add some butter.

Liver does not take very long to cook - don't make shoe leather.

You will turn it a couple of times until there is no visible blood coming through the flour. Until you get used to how long it takes, just cut a piece and see if it's cooked through. If it is all brown inside, it's done.

Put it on a warm plate back in the oven.

Step 6 - The Gravy

There should not be any fat left in the frying pan. If there is, you have used too much and you will need to pour it off - but don't clean the pan.

The spinach should be all cooked and there will be the spinach water in the bottom of the saucepan. Use a spatula or kitchen spoon to squeeze the spinach and get as much water as you can out of the spinach.

Pour this water into the frying pan.

There should be lots of water for gravy but, if not, you can use a little of the potato water, but don't make your gravy too salty.

If the potatoes are done, you should drain them at this point. You don't want them sitting in water as it will make the potatoes mushy.

OK, back to the gravy. Add a teaspoonful (5 mL) of Bovril™ or an OXO™ cube to the spinach water and heat to simmer as you stir the water and try to incorporate as much of the goodness on the fry pan as you can.

I also like to put in a couple of shakes of Worcestershire Sauce.

Mix up a couple of teaspoonsful (5g) of cornstarch in a small measuring cup. Add the water to the cornstarch very slowly and only use just enough to make the mixture pourable.

As you stir the gravy, slowly add the cornstarch until the gravy is the consistency of honey. When it is thick enough - stop.

Step 7 - Whip the Potatoes

Follow my previous directions and whip up the mashed potatoes. It's a good idea to hold the saucepan in the sink as you do this. Sometimes I over-crank my whipping action and send potato over the side of the saucepan.

Step 8 - Plate It

This is a guide to gourmet style liver and onions, so we need to consider how we are going to plate it.

This is a fairly big meal so you should start with a good-sized plate - you don't want to crowd everything together. You have white potatoes, brown meat and gravy plus dark green spinach, so a red, yellow or even blue plate might work well.

There are so many ways to arrange the food on the plate and nothing is wrong, but, you want to make it as attractive as possible. The following is just a suggestion, feel free to arrange it anyway you think looks good.

You want to get some height to the center of your plate, so you might start by placing some whipped potatoes in a line across the diameter of the plate. Not exactly in the center, you want one side of the potatoes bigger than the other.

Now place one or two strips of liver on the larger side of the potatoes. On the other side, put two or three strips of bacon. Drop the onion rings along the potatoes letting them fall on both the liver and the bacon.

Place a scoop of spinach on the liver side of the plate towards the plate's rim.

Drizzle gravy on the liver and the plate towards the spinach. On the bacon side, in the center of the empty space, put a small teaspoonful of yellow mustard.

Wine

This is a very rich, hearty meal and you need a wine that can compete and not get lost. Look for a full-bodied red wine like Burgundy, Pinot Noir or Merlot.

Recap

Bacon

Cook the bacon first in a large frying pan (you'll use the same pan to cook the liver). You'll need about 2-3 pieces of bacon per person.

Put the cooked bacon on some paper towel (on a plate) and keep warm in the oven (about 200° F (100° C, Gas Mark ½).

Onions

Cook the onions (sliced into thin rings) in the bacon fat until translucent.

Put the cooked onions on some paper towel (on a plate) and keep warm in the oven (about 200° F (100° C, Gas Mark ½).

Note: you should have the dinner plates warming in the oven at the same time.

Potatoes and Spinach

Cook the potatoes and the spinach at approximately the same time, so they will be ready together.

The potatoes are done when you can easily stick a fork in them.

Pour off the water and once the liver is cooked, whip the potatoes before serving.

Use about one 10 ounce (285g) package of baby spinach for each person. It cooks down quite a bit.

The spinach should be well rinsed but don't put any extra water in the saucepan.

Cook on a low heat so you don't burn the bottom leaves. Halfway through cooking, stir the spinach leaves on the top to the bottom of the pan.

Once the spinach is cooked, squeeze all the excess water out of the spinach and use that water to make the gravy.

Liver

Buy beef liver in $^3/_8$" (1 cm) slices if possible. Remove all fat, sinews and holes.

Dredge the liver in all purpose flour so that it is completely covered.

While the potatoes and spinach are cooking, fry the floured liver pieces in the bacon grease.

Liver doesn't take very long to cook. It is done once the liver is brown right through. Don't over cook it or you will make it tough.

Remove the liver from the frying pan and place in a warm oven with the bacon and onions.

Gravy

There shouldn't be any grease left in the frying pan. If there is, pour it off leaving any bits from frying the liver.

Pour the spinach water into the frying pan and heat. Add a beef bouillon cube, or Bovril, and dissolve well. Be sure to scrape any bits off the bottom of the frying pan so they get incorporated into the gravy.

Thicken gravy with cornstarch.

Colemans™ Mustard

Prepare the Colemans mustard so it's ready when you plate the meal.

Plating

Now that everything is ready, remove the warmed dinner plates from the oven and plate each dish. Be sure not to crowd everything and put the gravy on last.

Instant Pot™ Mashed Potatoes

About the only part of this meal that can be cooked in the Instant Pot™ are the mashed potatoes. You can cook bacon in the Air Fryer but it makes a mess and we want the bacon fat to cook the onions and liver.

The best part of using the Instant Pot™ in this situation is that it is one less thing to think about. Once you click the button you can get on with the rest of the meal and the potatoes will be ready for you when you get to them.

Ingredients

4 tablespoons (60g) butter
2 pounds (900g) Yukon Gold or Russet potatoes, peeled and sliced ½ inch (1.25 cm) thick
2 teaspoons (10 mL) sea salt
¾ cup (180 mL) whole milk

Directions

1. Using Sauté mode, melt the butter in the Instant Pot™.
2. Add the potato slices, sprinkle with salt and toss the potatoes to cover with the salt and butter.
3. Turn off the Sauté mode.
4. Add the milk and stir.
5. Lock the lid, set on Manual Mode for 7 minutes on High Pressure.
6. Quick release the pressure.
7. Remove the inner pot and place on a heat-proof surface.
8. Mash the potatoes to the desired consistency. While you're mashing, the potatoes should absorb any of the liquid left in the pot.
9. Serve and enjoy!

SUNDAY ROAST

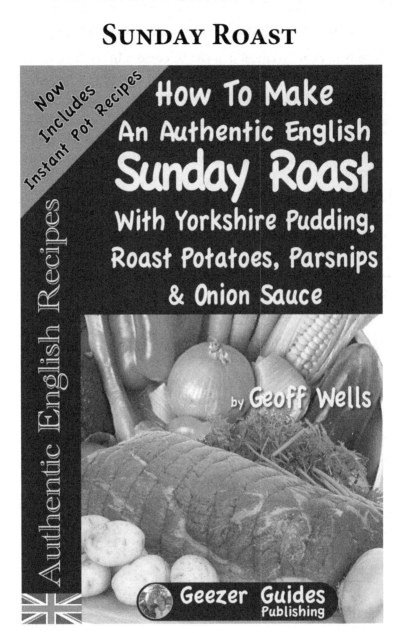

The Sunday Roast

The Sunday Roast is a tradition in England both at home and in the pubs. Visit any pub in England on Sunday and expect to see roast beef, pork or lamb on the menu - maybe all three.

But as good as pub food is you can do better by following these simple steps.

Selecting the meat.

Although the meat is the main focus of the meal it is the simplest part to cook. Roasting is just applying dry heat until the internal temperature reaches a certain level. Because you are using dry heat you need to purchase the most tender grade and cut you can afford. The cuts sold as roasts are the most tender but the grade can make a big difference in the outcome of your meal so buy Prime if possible or choose pork which is always tender.

Lamb

If you will be serving lamb then your choice is generally shoulder of lamb or leg of lamb. For some reason lamb is not as popular in North America as either beef or pork and that's a pity because you are missing a tender sweet treat. Lamb needs to be cooked slowly, if you try to rush it, it can be tough.

Personally I prefer lamb shoulder but the leg seems to be easier to get.

Prime and Choice grades are all you are likely to see for lamb. Either can be successfully roasted.

Pork

A pork roast is easy to find and you can use loin, picnic shoulder or the fancier crown roast. If you are cooking a crown roast place it in the roasting pan with the bones down for the first hour then turn it over and fill the cavity with stuffing and continue cooking until your meat thermometer registers 185°F (85°C).

Pork is uniformly tender and is not graded so any pork roast is fine.

Beef

Of course beef is the most popular and you have a range of cuts to choose from. Most popular roasts are rump and standing rib.

Choose Prime or Choice grades for roasting as the lower grades will not be sufficiently tender when cooked with dry heat.

How To Roast

Basically you stand the meat in a roasting pan and put it in the oven. Not rocket science but it's amazing what can go wrong. A friend of ours inadvertently tripped the self clean feature of the oven, the door locked and she cooked the roast for three hours at over 800°F. Understandably it was a little over done.

A probe type thermometer is a good investment. This is the type you insert into the roast so you can measure the temperature in the center. I will give you some cooking times per pound later on but there is really no substitute for a thermometer.

We used to use a large roasting pan and surround the meat with potatoes, parsnips, carrots and onions but now I prefer to cook the potatoes and parsnips separately.

So the bottom line is to preheat the oven to 350°F (175°C, Gas Mark 4) for pork, 300°F (150°C, Gas Mark 2) for beef and lamb. Put the roast in the middle of the roasting pan and surround it with carrots and onions sufficient to serve your guests.

Stick your thermometer probe in the meat so that the tip of the probe is in the center of the roast and not touching any bones. Place the pan in the oven so that you can see the thermometer dial through the oven door.

Oven Roasting Beef

Serve with horseradish sauce.

A beef roast will generally be between 2 and 4 pounds (1 to 1.8 Kg). The various cuts are Inside Round, Prime Rib, Sirloin Tip, Top Sirloin, and Tenderloin.

If you can find it and if you can afford it, choose grass fed beef. There is a tremendous difference in taste that is absolutely worth the price. Cows are supposed to eat grass not corn and grass fed cows are not injected with all the chemicals that the factory raised cattle are subjected to.

Seasoning

Make some shallow cuts as if you were slicing the roast and rub in some of you favorite seasonings. Try mixing a little olive oil, salt & pepper together with minced garlic, dried thyme, dried rosemary and a little lemon zest.

Searing

Searing is the process of sealing in the meat juices by subjecting the exterior to high heat. It can be done on the stove top using a frying pan or in the oven at 450°F (230°C, Gas Mark 8). In the oven sear for 7 minutes per pound but no more than 30 minutes total.

Beef Cooking Times

Lower the oven temperature to 325° F (160° C, Gas Mark 3) and cook for 18 to 22 minutes per pound or until the meat thermometer registers 125° F (52° C).

Cover your roast in foil and let it rest for 15 - 20 minutes before carving. It will continue to cook and the internal temperature will continue to rise until it is cut. Final temperatures are-

    145°F (63°C) medium-rare
    160°F (71°C) medium
    170°F (77°C) well done

Oven Roasting Lamb

Serve with mint sauce.

The cuts of lamb you see most often are leg and shoulder. The leg usually has the bone in and the shoulder is boneless. Leg is more expensive than the shoulder but the shoulder is tastier and easier to cook.

Seasoning

A rub of rosemary and garlic is recommended along with salt, pepper and olive oil.

Searing

Remove from fridge 1 hour before cooking

Broil the lamb for 5 minutes or until the top of the lamb leg looks seared and browned.

Flip the lamb over and put back under the broiler for 5 minutes or until the other side is seared.

Flip the lamb leg over again and rub the top with the chopped garlic and rosemary.

With the bone in, a leg of lamb will be 5 to 7 pounds

> 3 tablespoons (45 mL) olive oil
> Salt and freshly ground black pepper
> 6 cloves garlic
> 3 stems fresh rosemary
> Roasting Temperature: 325°F (165° C, Gas Mark 3)

Lamb Cooking Times

Rare: 125°F (52° C), (about 15 minutes per pound)

Medium-Rare: 130°F to 135°F (55°C to 57°C), (about 20 minutes per pound)

Medium: 135°F to 140°F (57°C to 60°C), (about 25 minutes per pound)

Well-Done: 155°F to 165°F (68°C to 74°C), (about 30 minutes per pound)

Select a roast that is at least 4 pounds (2 Kg).

Choose prime or choice grades so the meat will be tender. Leg of lamb is most commonly available but shoulder is also a good choice.

Oven Roasting Pork

Serve with apple sauce.

Select a roast that is at least 4 pounds (2 Kg).

Pork is uniformly tender and is, therefore, not graded.

Roast at 350°F (175°C, Gas Mark 4) (for about 40 minutes per pound (450g) or until the internal temperature reaches 185°F (85°C).

Seasoning

My favorite seasoning for a pork roast is Basil.

Combine 1 tablespoon (15 mL) of dried Basil with 2 - 3 tablespoons (30 - 45 mL) of olive oil and rub all over the pork roast.

Searing

A pork roast does not need to be seared.

Pork Cooking Times

Pork doesn't have rare, medium and well states - just properly cooked. It is important that pork be sufficiently cooked.

Cook it at 350°F (180°C, Gas Mark 4) for 40 minutes per pound (450g).

The internal temperature, when it is fully cooked, should be 185°F (85°C)

Oven Roasting Poultry

Serve with sage & onion stuffing

You might want to consider a simple roast chicken for your Sunday dinner. I'm not talking about the full blown Thanksgiving/Christmas Turkey experience which I detail in my book "How To Cook A Thanksgiving / Christmas Turkey Dinner". - (http://amzn.to/2sQptze). This is a much simpler affair where you replace the beef, lamb or pork with a chicken.

Seasoning

The seasoning goes inside for poultry where it also helps soak up the excessive amount of fat in the meat. See the "Sage & Onion Stuffing" section later on in this book.

Searing

No searing for poultry, in fact you need to cover wing tips and breast with tin foil so that they don't dry out or burn. Just remove the foil for the last half hour of cooking.

Poultry Cooking Times

Always use a thermometer inserted into the thigh - but not touching the bone.

The bird will continue to cook a little after you remove it from the oven but before you start to carve ensure that the thermometer reads at least 165°F (75°C).

Condiments

Mint Sauce (For Lamb)

One of my favorite things about a lamb roast is that I get to cover everything in mint sauce. If you have to buy it that's better than no mint sauce at all, but it is so easy to grow fresh mint and make your own.

It's best I say nothing about mint jelly.

Pick a few fresh mint leaves, then wash and finely chop them. Put the chopped leaves in a small container like a shot glass and cover with malt vinegar. Add a teaspoonful (5 mL) of sugar (or less) and stir. That's it. Just drizzle over the meat and anywhere else on your plate if you love fresh mint sauce.

AppleSauce (For Pork)

Jars of applesauce are easy to buy but your Sunday pork roast deserves better. Just finely chop a cooking apple like Bramley, Granny Smith or Spy, put in a small saucepan and add a little water - just a tablespoonful. Add some sugar or leave the tart apple taste. Boil for a few minutes until the apple is softened then serve warm.

If you own an Instant Pot you can also try the Instant Pot Applesauce Recipe later on in this book.

Horseradish Sauce (For Beef)

Store bought horseradish sauce is for wimps, even the stuff that claims to be "HOT" is mild compared to the fresh home grown variety. Of course if you don't like it, it makes no sense to ruin your meal just because it's the traditional condiment with beef.

For those of you that like horseradish, at least once in your life try the fresh homemade version. Horseradish is a root that is easy to grow or you can sometimes find it in a specialty grocery store. Use a vegetable peeler to remove the outer skin from an 8-10 inch (20-25 cm) long root.

Horseradish is way more potent than onions so don't touch your eyes without thoroughly washing your hands first. Even the fumes can be irritating so do your processing in a well ventilated area.

Put the chopped up root in a food processor with 2 tablespoonsful of water and process until well chopped. If there is too much liquid pour some off and add a tablespoonful of vinegar and a pinch of salt. Process again to combine the vinegar.

Put the mixture in a glass jar which you can refrigerate for 3 - 4 weeks.

Sage & Onion Stuffing (For Poultry)

Preparing a full Thanksgiving or Christmas dinner is more involved than the basic Sunday roast. I have included recipes for making stuffing bread and the actual stuffing below but if you want step by step Thanksgiving directions I urge you to look at my "How To Cook A Thanksgiving / Christmas Turkey Dinner". - (http://amzn.to/2sQptze)

Stuffing Bread

Ingredients

- 1 cup (240 mL) water
- 1 large egg
- 3 tablespoons (45 mL) olive oil
- ½ onion, chopped
- 2 teaspoons (10 mL) brown sugar
- ½ teaspoon (2.5 mL) salt
- ½ teaspoon (2.5 mL) black pepper, freshly ground
- 2 teaspoons (10 mL) poultry seasoning
- 1 teaspoon (5 mL) celery seeds
- 2½ cups (300g) flour
- 1½ teaspoons (7.5 mL) yeast
- ⅔ cup (100g) cornmeal

Method

Place ingredients in your bread maker in the order suggested by the manufacturer.

Select the white bread setting for a 2 pound (1Kg) loaf with a light crust. Press start.

After the bread has cooled slice it into ½ inch (1cm) thick slices and lay the slices out so they can get a little stale. You want the bread to be crumbly rather than moist. Cover the slices with a tea towel and leave them out overnight. You can also spread the slices on a cookie sheet and put the sheet in the oven. If they are not sufficiently dry in the morning just set the oven at 170°F (77°C) (lowest setting) and leave them for an hour.

Sage & Onion Stuffing

This recipe is enough for a 15 - 20 pound (7 - 9 Kg) turkey. You can alternatively stuff the neck cavity with sausage meat which adds some variety.

Ingredients

15 cups (750 g) of stuffing bread crumbs - (see recipe above)
1 medium to large onion
1 cup (225 g) melted butter
⅓ cup (5 g) fresh chopped sage (or 1 tablespoon (15 mL) dried sage)

Method

The size of your bread crumbs will effect the density of your stuffing. If you use very fine bread crumbs your stuffing will form a dense lump, if you use large pieces of bread your stuffing won't hold together. The best compromise is to use bread pieces that are a bit less than croûton size - less than quarter inch cubes. If you have done as I suggested and dried your slices of bread in the oven you can now tear the slices into small pieces. Take half-a-dozen pieces and rub them in the palm of your hands. They will crumble into perfect bread crumbs.

Add the fresh sage and chopped onion to your bread crumbs and mix well. Now add the melted butter and mix again. You don't want the mixture to be too wet as it is the job of the stuffing to absorb the juices from the turkey but you need enough butter so that the mixture holds together. Adjust the quantity of butter as required.

Fill both turkey cavities with the mixture and seal with skewers or use the plastic fastener that probably came with the turkey.

Yorkshire Pudding

Traditionally, in our house, Yorkshire Pudding was served with the Sunday roast. The roast came out of the oven to be carved and the Yorkshire mixture was poured into the roasting pan. It went back in the oven and was ready by the time the roast was carved.

There are no requirements that you do it that way but it does have the advantage of picking up all the wonderful flavours that are left on the bottom of the roasting pan.

The recipe for Yorkshire Pudding is the easiest thing in the world. Equal parts flour and milk (usually a cup each), an egg and a pinch of salt. If it doesn't rise properly, the next time try two or even three eggs but cut back on the milk as you don't want the batter too thin.

The secret to successful Yorkshire pudding is not in the recipe, it's in the method.

If you're planning to serve a Yorkshire, prepare the mixture early and let it get to room temperature. If you try to make it with milk cold from the fridge it is less likely to rise.

What most people think of when they think of Yorkshire pudding is a light, crispy and delicious sort of pancake. But that is not actually the original Yorkshire pudding. I had "real" Yorkshire pudding once and it is more like a suet pudding than what we think of today.

Ingredients

    1 cup flour (120g) (either self-raising flour or all-purpose flour with 1 teaspoon (5 mL) of baking powder added)
    1 egg (up to 3)
    1 cup (240 mL) milk
    ¼ teaspoon (1.25 mL) salt

Method

Mix well and allow to rest at room temperature for a couple of hours.

Pre-heat oven to 450°F (230°C, Gas Mark 8) (after roast has been removed).

Use either the roasting pan or a muffin tin with sufficient fat (about ¼" or .5 cm) in the bottom.

Heat pan and fat to 450°F (230°C, Gas Mark 8) and carefully add the Yorkshire Pudding batter.

Bake in the hot oven for 20-25 minutes. Watch it carefully through the glass window of the oven. Avoid opening the oven door while it is cooking.

Success Is In The Details

OK, let's refine my earlier recipe just a bit. Start with 1 cup of self-raising flour. Outside of England you're probably saying "What?". Self-raising flour is available in the US and Canada, but you might have to look for it in the specialty or imported section.

If you can't find it, don't worry about it. Just add a teaspoonful of baking powder to your regular, all-purpose white flour.

Beat a large egg and most of 1 cup (240 mL) of milk in a large measuring cup or bowl. Don't add all the milk because that might make the mixture too thin. Gradually add the flour making sure you don't get any lumps.

You are looking for a batter that is thicker than water but not as thick as honey. When you pour it into the pan you want it to spread to all sides but only just. After you've made a few you will know what I mean. So add as much of the remaining milk as you need to make the batter the right consistency

The idea here, as in all the books of this series, is not to blindly follow a recipe but to know why you are doing something and to make adjustments as you go.

Salt

Don't forget to add some salt. ¼ teaspoon (1.25 mL) is enough, but you need it as part of the chemistry of cooking.

Rest

As I said before, mix it early and let it sit on the counter so it will reach room temperature. It will still work if you don't but it will rise better if the batter is not fridge cold.

Cook It

It will take 20 - 30 minutes to cook in a 450°F - 500°F (230°C, Gas Mark 8 - 260°C, Gas Mark 10) oven so you should put it in the oven after everything else is done. Keep an eye on it so it doesn't burn, but don't open the oven - just peek through the glass.

Once it's done it gets cold very quickly so you want to put it on the plates just before bringing them to the table.

Two Ways

As I said in the beginning, your Yorkshire can be cooked in the roasting pan, which is the preferred way, or you can use a muffin pan and make individual Yorkshires, which Americans call Popovers. The advantage of cooking individual servings is that you obviously have more control over the serving size and they are less likely to fail.

Sometimes, if everything is not just right, a Yorkshire in the pan won't rise as much as it should. It can happen with Popovers, too, but it's harder to tell.

Hot Oven

Before you're ready to cook your Yorkshire, your roast pan or muffin pan should be up to about 450° F (230° C) or more. There should be a ¼" (.5 cm) of fat in the pan or each muffin cup.

The preference is for fat from the roast but any high temperature oil will work. Canola or Safflower oils are inexpensive and can take the high temperature without smoking too much.

When you're ready, remove the pan with the hot oil from the oven and put it firmly on top of the stove. Use premium quality oven mitts. You don't want to drop hot oil.

Pour the Yorkshire mix evenly into the pan. It will start cooking immediately but you want to get the pan bottom covered if you can.

Get the pan back in the oven as quickly and safely as you can.

I hope you have an oven with a glass you can see through because you need to resist the temptation to open the oven door to check on its progress.

Continue plating your meal and add the Yorkshire just before bringing the plates to the table.

Roast Potatoes & Parsnips

It just wouldn't be a Sunday roast without roast potatoes and parsnips. Some Americans call parsnips white carrots but they are only like carrots in appearance, the taste is much different. They have a sweet nutty flavour I'm sure you will enjoy.

Fresh carrots and parsnips are crisp not squishy. Be particularly careful when buying parsnips because they don't sell as quickly as carrots and some stores will keep them on the shelf well after they should be thrown away. If you can buy them loose so much the better but if you have to buy a bag look for parsnips about 1 - 1½ inches (2.5 - 3.5 cm) in diameter at the top.

Use a potato peeler to peel the parsnips then cut them in half so that you have a fat end and a thin end.. Cut the fat end in quarters lengthwise so you end up with five pieces all about the same length and thickness. Please don't take this too literally, I'm just trying to describe a process but it is not critical.

There are more than five hundred varieties of potatoes each with it's own taste and texture. You will never find that much choice in any store but you should try to choose the potato with the characteristics you need for the way you plan to cook them.

For roasting potatoes choose a low starch variety like King Edward, Red or New. You can also use a medium starch potato like Yukon Gold. Baking potatoes get too soft and tend to fall apart when you roast them.

Peel the potatoes and cut them into four to eight pieces depending on the size of the potato.

Allow at least one large potato per person and then add a couple of extra.

Any leftovers make great fry-up.

Parsnips generally come in a 2 or 3 pound (1.0 - 1.5 Kg) bag, so cook the entire bag.

Crispy Roast Potatoes & Parsnips

I like mine to be crispy so I cook them in a separate Pyrex™ dish which goes in the oven with the Yorkshire pudding.

For this method boil the parsnip and potato pieces in salted water for 5 - 10 minutes.

Drain them and pat them dry. Water will cause the hot oil to spit and will shorten the life of the oil if you plane to reuse it.

In a separate Pyrex™ dish (I use a 9" x 13" dish, (23cm x 33cm)) add sufficient oil (about ¼", 0.6 cm) and heat the dish in the hot oven like you do for the Yorkshire Pudding.

Using a kitchen spoon place the pieces in the Pyrex™ dish that contains the hot oil. Turn the pieces in the oil so that they are well covered.

Put the dish in the very hot oven with the Yorkshire pudding. They are done when they are golden brown which will be about the same time as the Yorkshire. About 20-25 minutes.

Pan Roasted Potatoes & Parsnips

As I said earlier you can put the potatoes and parsnips around the roast or you can cook them separately. The result will be slightly different depending on your method. If you put them around the roast they will absorb some of the meat juices, which is great, but they won't get crispy.

It's as simple as arranging them around the roast about an hour before the roast will be done.

Air Fryer Roast Potatoes & Parsnips

If you own an Air Fryer you can use it to roast your potatoes and parsnips. I've included the instruction in a separate section later on in the book.

Onion Sauce

Onion sauce is something that is always served with the Sunday roast - at least it was at our house. It is super easy to make yet I never seem to make enough at dinner parties we have had, because everyone asks for more.

Start by peeling and cutting up ordinary white onions. Chop them lengthwise but as thin as you can - about ⅛ inch (.3 cm). One 3 inch (7.5 cm) diameter onion is enough for two servings so judge how much you need accordingly. If in doubt make more because the leftovers will keep in the fridge for several days.

Put the chopped onion in a small saucepan and 'just' cover with water. Don't drown them because you will use this water for gravy and you don't want to dilute the flavour.

Bring the water to a boil and cook for 10 - 15 minutes or until the onions are done. Pour off and save the water.

Now add enough milk to 'just' cover and ½ teaspoonful (2.5 mL) of salt to the cooked onions and heat the milk. Don't let it boil or it will boil all over your stove.

In a cup or measuring cup mix up some cornstarch. How much will depend on how much onion sauce you're making but 2 teaspoonsful (10 mL) should be enough for the one large onion in the example. Cornstarch should be mixed with as little water as possible - just enough to make it pourable.

When the onion milk mixture is very hot, but not boiling, slowly stir in the cornstarch until the milk thickens and you have onion sauce.

Green Veg & Carrots

Fresh peas, brussels sprouts or scarlet runner beans are the green veggie of choice but go ahead with broccoli, cabbage or whatever else is in season.

Whichever green vegetable you choose, remember, it only needs to be fork tender. Don't cook it to death, boiling for ten minutes is generally sufficient. Also, only use enough water to 'just' cover. You will be using the water to make your gravy, so you don't want to dilute the goodness.

Steaming

A better method to cook vegetables is to steam them. Pick up a metal or silicon steaming insert for your saucepan - just a couple of dollars at Walmart™. Put an inch (2.5cm) of water in the bottom of the saucepan with the vegetables on top of the steamer. Put the lid on the saucepan and boil for 10 minutes

Scarlet Runner Beans

These are very popular in England but never seen in North American stores. This is surprising because the Scarlet Runner is native to North America. The seeds are available in North America and some gardeners grow them just for their bright red flowers.

They grow very well in cool climates so are an ideal crop for Canada and the Northern States. The Scarlet Runner Bean is my personal favorite green vegetable and I could easily eat a plateful and nothing else.

Carrots

Carrots are a very underrated and unappreciated vegetable because they always seem to be overcooked - at least in my experience. Add a few to your steamer basket and stop cooking when you can insert a fork into them - they're done!

Gravy

After you remove the cooked Yorkshire pour off any excess oil that may be in the roasting pan.

Scrap the bottom of the roasting pan to release any drippings or meat.

Add the onion water to the roasting pan and heat, on top of the stove, stirring to incorporate any juices from the roasting pan.

Add some of the green vegetable water to make the amount of gravy you want.

Ideally you will now add Bisto™ for truly authentic British gravy or you can add Bovril™ or a crumbled OXO™ bouillon cubes.

Add a couple of shakes of Worcestershire sauce. heat to almost boiling and thickened with cornstarch.

Don't forget to add any juice that leaks from the roast as you carve it.

Dessert

For a truly authentic English dessert serve whatever you like just so long as it's covered with Birds Custard. This is a family joke, and I couldn't resist, sorry mum.

Actually this is time for a plug for some of my other books in this series.

I'm sure you've heard of English Trifle but you may not of heard of Fool's - at least not the ones you have for dessert. You'll find recipes for both in Volume 2, "How to Make Sherry Trifle and British Fools"

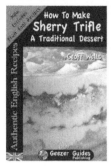

https://ebooks.geezerguides.com/how-to-make-sherry-trifle-and-british-fools-traditional-english-deserts/

You should also check our Volume 10, "How to Make Spotted Dick & Other Suet Puddings", which is full of all kinds of delicious authentic English desserts.

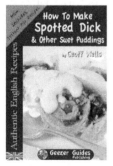

https://ebooks.geezerguides.com/how-to-make-spotted-dick-other-suet-puddings/

AND NOW FOR SOMETHING COMPLETELY DIFFERENT - PANCAKES (CRÊPES)

English pancakes are completely different to North American pancakes. North American pancakes are thick and doughy, eaten with butter and syrup and sometimes as a side order with eggs and bacon.

English pancakes are traditionally eaten only on Shrove Tuesday, are thin, crisp and eaten with sugar and lemon. In North America they are called crêpes.

This all relates to a book on Yorkshire pudding because they both use exactly the same batter. Except the batter is a bit thinner.

To make English pancakes heat a lightly greased frying pan to 325°F (165°C) and pour in enough batter to just cover the bottom of the pan. You will need to tip and turn the pan to get the batter to cover the whole bottom. Keep it thin.

Cook until the pancake releases from the pan and you can move it about.

Flip the pancake and sprinkle a teaspoonful of (5 mL) sugar over the cooked surface. Then add two teaspoonsful (10 mL) of lemon juice on top of the sugar.

When the pancake releases roll it up like you would roll up a carpet.

Pop it onto a warm plate and place in a warm oven 200°F (100°C, Gas Mark ½) while you make some more.

You can speed up the process by using more than one frying pan. It's a bit slow but makes a nice change for a Sunday lunch.

Check YouTube™ for pancake races that take place in English villages on Shrove Tuesday. It's a regular footrace with the twist that competitors carry a frying pan and flip their pancakes as they race.

Toad in the Hole

No Brits don't eat toads (most of them, anyway).

The "toads" in this dish are pork sausages cooked in the oven and surrounded by Yorkshire pudding.

Lay your pork sausages in the roasting pan then put them in the hot 450° F - 500° F (230°C, Gas Mark 8 - 260°C, Gas Mark 10) oven to start cooking. Take them out after 10 minutes and check the amount of oil in the pan. Add enough oil to bring the level to no more than ¼ inch (.5 cm). If you added oil put the pan back in the oven to bring the oil up to heat.

Yorkshire must be added to smoking hot oil so once you have it up to temperature go ahead and pour in the batter as I described above. Be very careful the pan is hot and you will feel it through cheap oven mitts.

When the Yorkshire is golden brown on the edges it is done. Remove from the oven and serve with mashed potatoes, gravy and onion sauce, (see the method above)

Instant Pot Roasting

Although cooking your Sunday roast in a pressure cooker may not really seem like "roasting", it still produces an amazing tender and tasty roast.

Technically, roasting is a dry heat process so it is wrong to call cooking in the Instant Pot, roasting but it definitely gets the job down and in a very short time.

Not only that, because you need to have some liquid in the pressure cooker for the pressure to build, you'll have liquid to make your gravy that's well-seasoned and tasty, too.

Times will vary slightly depending on the kind of meat you are cooking but the size of the "chunk" is the biggest factor. Cubes of stewing beef will cook faster than a single roast.

To be sure you can always insert a meat thermometer to check for doneness.

Beef
Rare [52°C, 125°F] • Medium [63°C, 145°F] • Well [71°C, 160°F]

Lamb
Medium [63°C, 145°F] • Well [71°C, 160°F]

Pork
No less than [85°C, 185°F]

Chicken & Turkey
No less than [75°C, 165°F]

Ingredients

3 - 4 lbs (2 to 2.5 Kg) roast (I urge you to pay the extra for animals raised in ethical conditions. Also grass fed beef is worth every penny for the wonderful taste)

Herbs to taste, such as thyme, rosemary, basil, etc. (I often use Herbes de Provence)

12 ounces (350 mL) vegetable broth (or chicken or beef)

2 cloves of garlic, halved

3 - 4 large carrots, peeled and chunked

2 medium onions, quartered

1 or 2 bouillon cubes, packets or liquid

Method

1. Rub the roast well with the herbs of your choice and let it sit for an hour or so.
2. Pour the broth into the Instant Pot, add the garlic, place the trivet in the bottom and place the roast on the trivet.

3. Close the lid, select the Manual setting and set the time for 35 minutes.
4. When cooking time is up, use Natural Pressure Release for 10 minutes, then release the pressure.
5. Use a meat thermometer to check the internal temperature at the thickest part - but not touching a bone.
6. Add the carrots and onions to the Instant Pot, close the lid, select the Manual setting for 5 minutes.
7. When cooking time is up, use Natural Pressure Release for 10 minutes and then release pressure.
8. Remove the carrots and onions to a warm serving dish and place in a 170°F, (77°C) oven to keep warm.
9. Check the temperature again but it should be done. (remember it will continue to cook slightly until you carve it)
10. Remove the roast and allow it to sit for 5-10 minutes before carving.
11. Add an appropriate bouillon flavor cube, packet or liquid to the broth for the type of meat you are cooking.
12. Place a tablespoonful of cornstarch into a small cup and stir in just enough water to make it pourable.
13. Click the Sauté button on the Instant Pot to bring the broth to a simmer and slowly stir in the liquid cornstarch.
14. Stop adding the cornstarch when the gravy is the consistency of honey.

Air Fryer
Roast Potatoes and Parsnips

Roast potatoes and parsnips are a mainstay for English Sunday Roast Dinners. In England, parsnips are quiet common but not so much in certain areas of North America. You might even find that they are called "white carrots". However, they don't taste like carrots at all. When roasted, parsnips have a wonderful, nutty flavor. If you haven't tried them, you should.

Notes:

1. Be sure to use either Russet or Yukon Gold potatoes as they work best and make tasty roast potatoes.

2. Most recipes will tell you to peel the potatoes, I don't. Why? For a few or reasons: there's really no need to; most of the nutrition is in the peel, so why waste it; I think they taste better with the skins left on.

3. Make sure to cut the parsnips so that they are relatively the same size and thickness. They will cook much more evenly that way.

Ingredients

    2 - 3 medium Russet or Yukon Gold potatoes, scrubbed
    3 - 4 medium parsnips, peeled

Method

1. Cut the well scrubbed potatoes into chunks.
2. Cut the peeled parsnips into 2 inch (5 cm) pieces. Halve, or quarter, the thicker sections so that all the pieces are about the same length and thickness.
3. Soak the potatoes and parsnips in cold water for at least ½ hour.
4. Drain them and dry thoroughly.
5. Pre-heat the air fryer to 400° F (200°C).
6. Place the potatoes and parsnips in a shallow bowl and drizzle them with the olive oil. Then toss to make sure they are evenly coated. Optionally, you can spray them with olive oil using an olive oil mister. If you have no idea what I'm talking about take a look at this page on Amazon. http://amzn.to/2wQojJc

7. Place the parsnips ONLY in the basket and cook for 8 minutes.

8. Remove the basket. Shake well. Add the potatoes and return the basket to the air fryer. Cook for 10 minutes more.
9. Remove the basket. Shake well. Return the basket to the air fryer and cook for an additional 10 minutes. Both the potatoes and parsnips should be cooked through and nicely browned.
10. Serve immediately.

INSTANT POT APPLESAUCE

Applesauce is a great addition to any pork roast Sunday dinner. This is an easy recipe to make your own using the Instant Pot.

You'll find lots of applesauce recipes that tell you to peel the apples, I don't. Why? There are lots of nutrients in apple's skin and flavor, too!

Some recipes will also suggest sweetening the applesauce, I don't. Why? Apples are naturally sweet, there's no need to add additional sweeteners.

INGREDIENTS

>6 - 8 medium to large apples (Granny Smith, Gala, McIntosh, Fuji, etc.), well washed
>1 cup (240 mL) water
>1 teaspoon (5 mL) lemon juice (freshly squeezed, if possible)

METHOD

1. Cut the well-washed apples into halves and then quarters. Remove the core and seeds then quarters into 2" (5 cm) chunks.
2. Place the apples in the Instant Pot along with 1 cup (240 mL) of water and 1 teaspoon (5 mL) lemon juice.
3. Close the Instant Pot lid and choose the Manual setting for 8 minutes. Be sure the steam vent is sealed.
4. Once the cooking cycle is complete, let the pressure release naturally for 2 - 3 minutes and then release the pressure.
5. Using an electric mixer or immersion blender to attain applesauce consistency. Alternately, you can place the cooked apples in a food processor.
6. Allow the applesauce to cool somewhat and then put it in clean, sterilized (running them through the dishwasher should be enough) mason jars and refrigerate.

Note: Homemade applesauce will be okay in the fridge for about a week. It also freezes well and you can keep it in the freezer for up to a year.

English Breakfast

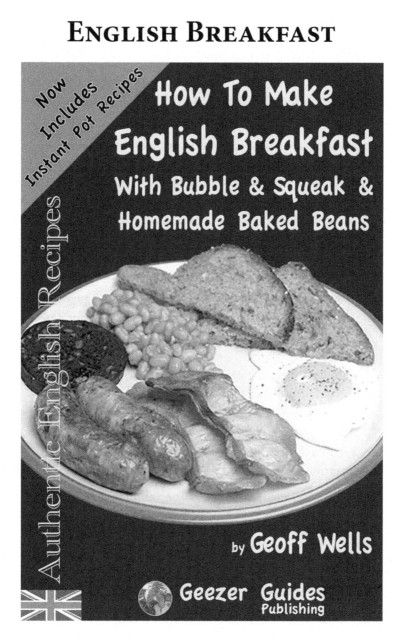

How To Make An English Breakfast

The Scots may have their porridge but Brits have their English Breakfast.

This is a breakfast you feed a man that is going to work on the farm all day or out on the fishing boats. Lots of protein to fuel your body for a day of hard work.

Most of us don't have hard, physically demanding jobs anymore but an English Breakfast can also be an English Brunch. It makes for a great mid-morning meal on a weekend when you have time to savor the delicious flavors. Have your yogurt and coffee during the week when that's all the time you have to eat before rushing off to the office. But, on the weekend, kick back and enjoy an old world pleasure.

Ingredients

These are the ingredients of the full English Breakfast. You won't necessarily include everything all the time. Just mix and match what you like.

Eggs

It's hard to imagine without the eggs but I guess you could. Eggs are really first on your ingredient list but the last thing you cook.

Meat

An English breakfast usually comes with a selection of meat. Not huge portions, just a variety of small pieces so that you can enjoy the different tastes.

Select from bacon, sausage, ham, liver, kidney and blood pudding*.

*Blood Pudding.

Blood pudding is a favorite with British vampires and actually tastes pretty good. If you can get past the name you will find it tastes like a premium sausage. It is popular all over Europe and Scandinavia.

In the US it is called Black Pudding or Black Sausage but it's still made with blood.

Fried Bread

When I was growing up in England, my mother used to maintain a "drippings basin". This was, essentially, a basin (ceramic bowl) into which she poured the fat that dripped from the Sunday roast. As it cooled it hardened and was available anytime we needed to fry something.

What made it different to the lard or cooking oil of today is the fact that it had flavor.

Fried bread is just that - bread fried in dripping until it is crisp.

You can get close by frying your bread in the bacon fat but be sure to pour off any of the water that comes out of bacon today when you first start to cook it.

Bubble & Squeak

Bubble & Squeak is made from leftover, already cooked, potatoes (bubble) and cabbage (squeak). So, the night before, just cook a little extra and put it aside in the fridge.

Some people have the idea that Bubble & Squeak is just warmed up potatoes and cabbage but it is much more. The two flavors are combined to create a third, totally different, flavor.

Start by finely chopping both ingredients. The potato will chop easily in the frying pan but pay particular attention to the cabbage. You don't want any large pieces.

You should have roughly equal amounts of potato and cabbage, which you put in a lightly greased frying pan together.

With a spatula turn and chop the mixture to make sure everything is well mixed together. Turn up the heat and put a little butter in the pan so you can lightly fry the mixture. Separate and shape into two pancakes.

The goal is to make the pancakes brown and crispy on the outside. There is nothing in the mixture to hold the ingredients together so the job you did of finely chopping the cabbage will determine how well the pancake stays together.

Use a large spatula the size of the pancake to turn them so they don't fall apart.

Fried Tomato With Marmite™

There are Marmite™ lovers™ and Marmite™ haters, no one is neutral when it comes to Marmite™. In Canada you can usually find it in the spices section of larger grocery stores. In the US, if you find it at all, it will be in with the imported foods. If you're an Aussie, sorry you'll just have to eat Vegemite™.

Check Wikipedia for a similar product in your part of the world.

Whatever you use just drop two ¼ teaspoonsfuls (1.25 mL) in the frying pan and cover with the two cut halves of a fresh tomato. I like mine just warm but you may want to cook it longer.

Baked Beans

The final component of an Authentic English Breakfast is baked beans.

So many things have change over the years, many not for the best. And baked beans is one of them.

50 years ago the beans were so tightly packed in the can you had to spoon them out. Now you get half a can of juice and a lot less beans.

The only way to get really good baked beans today is to make your own.

We usually had Heinz™ 57 Baked Beans in Tomato Sauce but I don't have that recipe. Fortunately my Canadian wife is a very talented cook and has come up with a recipe that tastes even better. She also has a family recipe, of her own, that uses molasses so I will share that with you to.

I'm also including the [Instant Pot version](#) for those of you that have one. (see Page 103)

Traditional English-Style Baked Beans

A tomato-based style of baked beans is generally the traditional type served with an English Breakfast.

Ingredients

    3 tablespoon (45 mL) salt
    8 cups (1.9 L) water
    2 cups (450g) dried white navy beans
    2 tablespoons (30 mL) olive oil
    1 medium onion, chopped
    2 cloves garlic, minced
    1 small carrot, peeled and finely chopped
    1 stalk celery, finely chopped
    1 bay leaf
    4 cups (900g) canned diced tomatoes
    2 tablespoons (30 mL) Worcestershire sauce
    2½ tablespoon tomato paste
    1 teaspoon (5 mL) balsamic vinegar
    1 tablespoon (15 mL) dark brown sugar

Method

1. In a large bowl or saucepan, dissolve the salt in 8 cups of water, add the beans and soak for at least 8 hours or overnight.
2. Drain and rinse the beans. Place them in a large saucepan and cover with fresh water.
3. Bring to a boil, skimming off any foam that is created. Boil for 4 minutes, then turn off, cover and let them sit for 1 hour.
4. In a small saucepan, heat the olive oil. Add the onion, garlic, carrot and celery. Sauté for 3 - 4 minutes.
5. In a large, oven-safe, pot, combine the beans, sautéed items and the rest of the ingredients. Stir well.
6. Cover and bake at 250°F (130°C, Gas Mark ½) for 2-3 hours.

Be sure to check that the beans don't dry out while they're in the oven. If they appear dry add a little water or broth and stir.

Homemade Baked Beans With molasses

Ingredients

- 2 cups (450g) dry navy beans
- 5 cups (1.2 L) water
- 1 1/2 (7.5 mL) teaspoons salt
- 1 cup (150g) onion, chopped
- 8 ounces (225g) salt pork
- 2 cups (475 mL) water
- ½ (120 mL) cup molasses
- ¼ cup (45g) brown sugar
- ½ (2.5 mL) teaspoon pepper
- ½ (2.5 mL) teaspoon salt

Method

1. Soak the beans in water overnight for at least for 12 hours.
2. Drain and combine the beans with 5 cups of water (1.2 L) and 1 ½ teaspoons (7.5 mL) salt.
3. Bring to a boil then reduce the heat, cover and simmer for 30 minutes.
4. Drain again and pour half of the beans into a greased 3 quart (2.8 L) baking dish
5. Sprinkle the beans with the cup of chopped onion.
6. Score the rind of the pork and place it on the layer of beans.
7. Add the remaining beans making a second layer on top of the pork.
8. Combine the remaining water, molasses, brown sugar salt and pepper then pour it over the beans.
9. Cover and bake 6 to 7 hours at 250°F (130°C, Gas Mark ½).
10. Add more water if required.
11. Bake uncovered for the last 30 minutes.
12. Makes 6 servings.

ENGLISH BREAKFAST RECIPE RECAP

You probably don't need a recipe but here is a quick recap of the ingredients and method for making an English Breakfast.

INGREDIENTS FOR TWO SERVINGS

 4 eggs
 4 slices of bacon
 2 pork breakfast sausages
 2 small pieces of ham
 2 small pieces of liver, floured
 2 small pieces of kidney
 2 slices of blood pudding
 1 cup (240 mL) leftover boiled potatoes
 1 cup (240 mL) leftover cabbage
 1 cup (240 mL) baked beans
 2 slices bread
 8 small mushrooms

METHOD

1. Put the bacon and sausage in a large frying pan over medium heat.
2. If water comes out of the bacon or sausage, pour it off and continue to cook.
3. Dust the liver and kidney with flour and add to the hot bacon fat.
4. When the meat is done, divide on two plates and place in warm oven.
5. Put the bread slices in the remaining fat and cook until brown and crisp. If there is not enough fat add some butter to the pan. When the fried bread is done add to the plates in the oven.
6. Put the chopped up potato and cabbage in the pan and form two pancakes. Cook on a high heat until brown and crispy. Add butter if required.
7. Your frying pan will now most likely have meat juices and bubble & squeak stuck on the bottom. If you try to fry the eggs in it they will stick. Either wipe the pan with paper towel or use a different pan for the eggs.

FRYING EGGS

Your lightly greased, clean frying pan should be at 350°F (175°C). before you add any eggs. The eggs should start to cook immediately. Many people make the mistake of adding eggs to a cold pan and then bringing it up to heat. This will make your eggs rubbery. If your pan is too hot the edges of your eggs will be burnt and crisp.

The fresher the egg is, the less likely the white is to spread. If your egg seems watery and runs it is less fresh - not bad, just not fresh.

When the eggs are done how you like them, add to the plates and serve with baked beans.

Mushrooms

Cook the mushrooms last so the juice doesn't make the eggs stick to the pan. Don't overcook mushrooms, you can eat them raw if you want. They are frequently served raw in salads so don't think you have to cook them to death.

Separate the stems from the tops, then drop a pat of butter in the pan and when it sizzles add the mushrooms. After a couple of minutes flip the tops over and roll the stems around a bit.

Toast, Crumpets or Muffins

As an alternative to fried bread you can serve toast, crumpets or muffins. If you're still hungry there is marmalade and tea.

A Lighter British Breakfast

Admittedly the full British breakfast is a bit more than you need unless you have a hard physical lifestyle.

The truth is, it's mostly the tourist that eat it today, except on weekends.

It's a sad fact that the US food conglomerates are slowly taking over even the British breakfast with their salt and sugar laden packaged products.

Fortunately you can still get my two favorite cereals growing up, Shredded Wheat and Weetabix. Unfortunately neither is British; Shredded Wheat is American and Weetabix is from Australia.

We always think of Scotland when Oats or porridge is mentioned but porridge has been a British breakfast favorite for centuries. Although traditionally cooked on the stove and before that in an iron pot slung over the fire the latest method is to use an Instant Pot. I have included this method in the Instant Pot section.

My mother lived to one hundred and two and she ate porridge for breakfast almost every day.

Another breakfast favorite was a poached egg on an English muffin. Sure, you can bye something called an English muffin from the supermarket bakery but look at the ingredient list before you bye it. Did you spot the plaster of paris used as the dough enhancer.

Turn the page for the traditional recipe that I borrowed from my "How To Bake British Cakes, Crumpets, Buns & Biscuits"- Book 9 in this series.

English Muffins

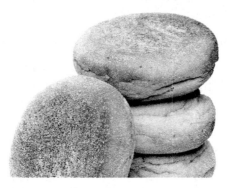

This is a traditional recipe that makes enough muffins for a large family. If you want less you can freeze the leftovers or look at the bread machine recipe in my Baking Book.

Ingredients

    1 cup (240 mL) milk
    2 tablespoons (25g) sugar
    2 teaspoons (10 mL) active dry yeast
    1 cup (240 mL) warm water
    ¼ cup (55g) butter, melted
    6 cups (720g) all purpose flour
    1 teaspoon (5 mL) salt
    cornmeal, for coating

Method

In a small saucepan, heat the milk over medium-low heat until it comes almost to the boil (small bubbles will form). Remove it from the heat and mix in the sugar until it dissolves. Set the saucepan aside and let the milk cool until it is lukewarm.

While the milk is cooling, put the warm water in a small bowl and sprinkle the yeast on top. Let is stand until it is frothy about 10 minutes.

> *Note: If the yeast does not froth then either the water is too hot or too cold or the yeast is no longer active. In that case, throw out the water/yeast mixture and start again.*

In a large bowl combine the milk, yeast mixture, melted butter, 3 cups (360g) of the flour and beat until smooth. Then add the salt and the remaining flour. Knead well until the dough is smooth and elastic.

Transfer the dough to a lightly greased bowl. Turn the dough to ensure it is lightly coated in the grease. Cover the dough with plastic wrap and move it to a warm place to rise until doubled in size - about one hour.

Note: The best place to let dough rise is in an oven with only the oven light turned on.

Once the dough has risen, remove the plastic wrap and turn it out onto a lightly floured surface. Punch down the dough and knead slightly. Roll the dough out to about ½ inch (1.25 cm) thick and cut out rounds with a cookie cutter (about 3 inches or 7.5 cm in diameter). Sprinkle a baking sheet with cornmeal and place the English muffins on the cornmeal. Then dust the tops of muffins with cornmeal as well. Loosely cover the muffins with plastic wrap and allow to rise for about ½ hour.

Note: The best place to let the muffins rise is in an oven with only the oven light turned on.

Heat a heavy skillet (preferably cast iron) over medium-low heat. Spray lightly with non-stick cooking spray.

Gently squeeze each muffin between your palms, being sure to keep them evenly flat, before placing in the hot skillet so they aren't too "puffy". Cook the muffins in the heavy skillet for about 5 to 7 minutes per side. When you turn the muffins, press down on them evenly with a spatula. The muffins will be golden brown on both sides when they are done.

Note: Squeezing the muffins before putting them in the pan and then pressing on them after you have turned them will help them maintain the traditional English muffin shape

You can split the muffins with a fork or serrated knife while they are still warm and serve immediately, or allow to cool on a wire rack.

These English muffins freeze well and can be thawed and toasted later.

Servings: 24

Poached Eggs on an English Muffin

Poached eggs are a satisfying alternative to fried eggs. Poaching an egg can take a little finesse, but the results are a perfectly cooked egg white with a lightly cooked, still liquid yolk.

Ingredients

>   2 - 4 eggs (depending on how many servings you want)
>   Water
>   Dash of white vinegar

Method

1. Fill a medium saucepan about ⅔ full of water.
2. Bring the water to a boil over medium-high heat.
3. Reduce the heat to bring the water to a bare simmer and add a dash of white vinegar.
4. Crack the egg into a small measuring cup or ramekin.
5. Gently tip the egg into the simmering water and cook for approximately 4 minutes. (The time will vary depending on your taste but 4 minutes should set the whites and leave the yolk still gooey and liquid).
6. Gently remove the poached eggs with a slotted spoon, let the water drain off.
7. Place each egg on a toasted English muffin and enjoy!

Instant Pot Traditional English-Style Baked Beans (No-soak method)

A tomato-based style of baked beans is generally the traditional type served with an English Breakfast. This Instant Pot no-soak recipe makes it easy to have Traditional English baked beans quickly.

Ingredients

- 2 tablespoons (30 mL) olive oil
- 1 medium onion, chopped
- 2 cloves garlic, minced
- 1 small carrot, peeled and finely chopped
- 1 stalk celery, finely chopped
- 2 cups (450g) dried white navy beans
- 2 cups (480 mL) vegetable broth or water
- 4 cups (900g) canned diced tomatoes
- 2 tablespoons (30 mL) Worcestershire sauce
- 3 tablespoons (45 mL) tomato paste
- 1 teaspoon (5 mL) balsamic vinegar
- 1 tablespoon (15 mL) dark brown sugar
- 2 teaspoons (10 mL) sea salt
- 1 bay leaf

Method

1. Select Sauté mode and allow the inner pot of your Instant Pot to heat up.
2. Add the olive oil and allow it to heat up
3. Add the onion, garlic, carrot and celery and sauté for 3-4 minutes.
4. Press Cancel to turn off Sauté mode.
5. Add the rest of the ingredients and stir well.
6. Close and lock the lid, ensuring the Pressure Valve is in the Sealing position.
7. Select the Bean/Chili Function and set the cooking time for 25 minutes.
8. When cooking time is complete, allow a full Natural Pressure Release. This means waiting until to Float Valve drops on it own.

    Tip: this can take up to 45 minutes.

    Tip: You can simple turn off your Instant Pot - press Cancel - and wait for the Float Valve to drop or you can let it go into Keep Warm mode, which it should do automatically. In Keep Warm mode the time will start counting up, ie you'll see L0:00, L0:01, L0:02, etc. It's counting up the minutes since the Bean/Chili function completed.)

9. Once the Float Valve has dropped, carefully open the lid, remove the bay leaf and give everything a good stir.
10. It may seem like there's a lot of liquid, but the beans will continue to absorb the sauce even after it has cooled down, so don't be tempted to thicken it.

> *Tip: The bake beans will taste much better if you let them sit for a day, allowing the flavors to mature. So, package them up and let them sit in the fridge for a day. You can have them cold or warm them up. Whatever your preference is.*

INSTANT POT HOMEMADE BAKED BEANS WITH MOLASSES

INGREDIENTS

2 cups or 1 lb. (450g) dry Navy beans (or Great Northern beans)
1 tablespoon (15 mL) extra virgin olive oil (optional, but recommended to keep the "foam" down when cooking the beans under pressure)
1 cup (150g) onion, chopped
4 ounces (110g) salt pork, sliced (bacon can be substituted)
½ cup (120 mL) molasses
¼ cup (45g) brown sugar
½ teaspoon (2.5 mL) pepper
1½ teaspoons (7.5 mL) salt

METHOD

1. Soak the beans in water overnight. Use enough water to cover the beans by at least two inches.
2. Discard the soaking water and rinse the beans.
3. Cover with 4 cups (950 mL) of fresh water, or more as needed and add the olive oil.
4. Add the remaining ingredients, stir and cook on the "Bean/Chilli" setting for 50 minutes.
5. When cooking time is up, use a Natural Pressure Release for 10 minutes, then release the pressure.
6. Test the beans to be sure they are consistently tender. If not, cook for another 5-10 minutes using the "Bean/Chilli" setting.
7. Once again, use a Natural Pressure Release for 10 minutes, then release the pressure.
8. Serve immediately or allow to cool then refrigerate or freeze for later use.

Makes 6 servings.

INSTANT POT POACHED EGGS

The Instant Pot method for poached eggs takes a lot of the guesswork out of the equation and the eggs never actually get immersed in the water.

INGREDIENTS

2-4 eggs (depending on how many servings you want)
1 cup (240 mL) water

METHOD

1. Place the water in the inner liner of your Instant Pot.
2. Spray individual silicone cups (one for each egg) with a non-stick cooking spray.
3. Crack one egg into each of the silicone cups and carefully place the cups on a stainless steel or silicone trivet.
4. Gently lower the trivet into the Instant Pot.
5. Close and lock the lid.
6. Select Steam mode and set the cooking time for 3 or 4 minutes.

   (We find we get a perfect poached egg at 3 minutes but your preference may vary. If you like a solid yolk, select 5 minutes.)
7. When the cooking time is complete, do a Quick Release to release all of the pressure.
8. Once all of the pressure is released, carefully open and remove the lid and gently lift the trivet out of the Instant Pot.
9. Carefully slide the poached eggs out of the silicone cups onto a toasted English muffin and enjoy!

INSTANT POT
ALMOND BUCKWHEAT PORRIDGE

This hearty breakfast is sugar-free, the sweetness is provided by the chopped prunes.

INGREDIENTS

- 1 cup (250g) buckwheat groats
- 2 cups (480 mL) whole milk
- 2 cup (480 mL) water
- ¼ cup (40g) raisins
- ¼ cup (30g) prunes, chopped and packed
- 1 teaspoon (5 mL) vanilla
- ¼ cup (20g) chopped almonds

METHOD

1. Rinse the buckwheat groats well and place them in the Instant Pot.
2. Add all the other ingredients and stir well.
3. Close and lock the lid and ensure that the valve is in the Sealing position.
4. Select Manual mode and set the cooking time for 6 minutes.
5. When the cooking time is complete allow a Natural Pressure Release (can take up to 20 minutes).
6. Once pressure is completely release, carefully remove the lid, stir the porridge and serve.

Instant Pot
Apple and Spice Steel Cut Oats

This is possibly the closest you can some to the taste of apple pie for breakfast.

Ingredients

½ cup (40g) steel cut oats
1 large apple, cored and chopped
1½ cups (360 mL) water
1½ (7.5 mL) teaspoons cinnamon
¼ teaspoon (1.25 mL) allspice (can substitute ground cloves)
¼ teaspoon (1.25 mL) nutmeg
1 tablespoon (15 mL) maple syrup or honey

Method

1. Add all items to the Instant Pot except the Maple Syrup and stir well.
2. Close and lock the lid, ensuring that the valve is in the Sealing position.
3. Select Manual mode and set the cooking time for 3 minutes.
4. Once cooking time is complete and allow a Natural Pressure Release.
5. Once pressure has been fully released, carefully open and remove the lid.
6. Stir in the maple syrup or honey and serve.

Devonshire Tea

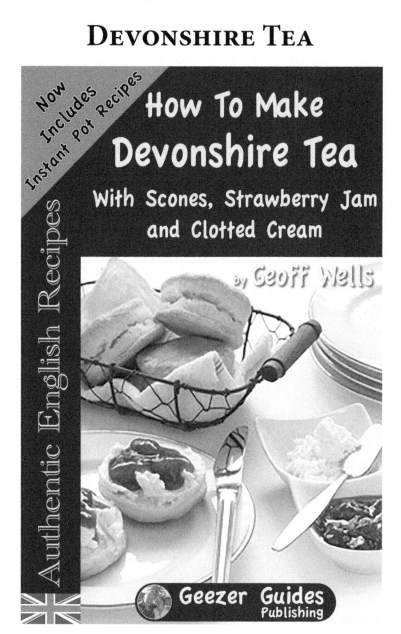

Introduction

Devon is one of my favorite areas in England. If I was to go back to live I would most likely choose Devon.

It is the South of England and enjoys the best climate with warm summer days and gentle sea breezes.

The coast is dotted with quaint fishing villages that have changed little in hundreds of years.

After a day of sightseeing by the time 4pm rolls around you'll probably be ready for a spot of tea. So it's good that the tea shops are so easy to find. Just squeeze yourself into one of the little tables and order a Devonshire Tea.

Devonshire tea is not a tea blend like Earl Grey or Orange Pekoe, it is a ritual performed everyday in small tea rooms throughout Southern England and particularly the County of Devon. A favorite pastime for both locals and tourists this tradition should definitely be on your to-do list whenever you visit Devon.

Real English tea with milk, fresh hot scones with homemade strawberry jam and mounds of clotted cream are what is on the menu at 4 o'clock in the afternoon.

This is an occasional indulgence so don't stress over the calories - just enjoy it.

How to Make Real English Tea

Order tea in any North American restaurant and the odds are good that you will get a pot of warm water and a tea bag on the side. This will make flavored water but it will not make tea.

There is probably nothing you can do about restaurant tea - besides avoiding it - but at least at home you can get it right.

Real Tea

Tea is an infusion made from leaves, loose tea is just chopped up leaves. The loose tea leaves go into the tea pot and when you pour the tea you use a tea strainer to catch the leaves before they get into the cup.

Tea Bags

There is nothing really wrong with the idea of tea bags. The problem is with the big food corporations that are always looking for ways to save a buck. Consequently the quality of the tea in the bags tends to be less than that of loose tea. Along with tea leaves you will often find tea dust.

Tea Balls

The compromise is to buy a tea ball that allows you to put loose tea in a small metal ball that has holes in it. This gives you the convenience of a tea bag and the quality of loose tea.

Of course you will still have the problem of finding loose tea in North America. Even in Canada it is not available in most supermarkets and your only option is to buy it from a specialty shop or online.

Making a Cuppa

Even if you are stuck with tea bags, you can do a much better job than any restaurant. An American restaurant is the worst place to get a decent cup of tea.

Boiling Water

Unlike coffee, which should never be boiled, tea requires boiling water to release the full flavor.

Warm the Pot

If you pour boiling water into a cold teapot much of the heat in the water will go towards warming the pot. To prevent this, either warm your teapot with hot tap water or use a little of the almost-boiling water from your kettle. Just pour some in the pot, swirl it around a bit and pour it out.

Add the Tea

Add your loose tea or tea bags to the warm pot. How much tea you use is, of course, a matter of personal taste depending on how strong you like it. Our rule was always one teaspoon per person plus one for the pot. But, like they say, "your mileage may vary".

If you are using tea bags, then one bag per person is probably a good place to start. But you can usually get enough for two cups from one tea bag if you use a pot.

Bring the Teapot to the Kettle

Water will stop boiling as soon as the heat source is removed. So, if you take the kettle from the stove to the pot, the water will not be boiling when you pour it on the tea. So the rule is - always take the pot to the kettle. When the water is at a rolling boil, pour it into the pot as quickly as you can.

Steep It

You need to allow the tea to sit and steep for 5 minutes to allow the flavors to get from the leaves and into the water.

Traditionally, at this point, you would cover the teapot with a tea cozy which was sort of a quilt made to fit the pot with openings for the spout and handle.

Milk, Sugar or Lemon

You can have your tea black or add various combinations of milk, sugar, honey or lemon. Don't put milk and lemon together as the lemon will curdle the milk. Another nice touch is to serve warm milk rather than milk from the fridge since the ice cold milk will cool the tea.

Recap

Warm the teapot using hot tap water or almost-boiling water from the kettle.

Swirl the hot water in the teapot and then pour it out.

Place the tea (loose, in a tea ball or tea bags) in the warmed pot.

Bring the teapot to the kettle and when the water is at a full rolling boil, pour it into the teapot as quickly as possible.

Steep for 5 minutes. If you have a tea cozy, put it on while the tea is steeping.

Enjoy your tea black or with whatever additions you like.

How To Make Scones

Ingredients

2 cups (240g) white all-purpose flour
3 teaspoons (15 mL) baking powder
½ teaspoon (2.5 mL) salt
2 tablespoons (25g) sugar
⅓ cup (65g) shortening
2 large eggs, slightly beaten
½ cup (120 mL) (approximately) whole milk or cream

Method

1. Pre-heat the oven to 425°F (220°C, Gas Mark 7).
2. In a large bowl, combine the flour, baking powder, salt and sugar. Mix well.
3. Cut in the shortening with a pastry blender until the mixture resembles a coarse corn meal.
4. In a separate measuring cup add enough milk to the slightly beaten eggs to make ¾ cup (175 mL). Mix well.
5. While stirring with a fork, add just enough of the liquid mixture to the flour mixture to make a soft dough.
6. Continue to stir until all of the flour disappears.
7. On a lightly floured surface, knead the dough for about 30 seconds
8. Either pat the dough down, or roll it out, to about ½ inch (1.25 cm) thick.
9. Cut into rounds with a cookie cutter. You should get 10 to 12 scones.
10. You can re-use any scraps left over from cutting the dough by reforming and cutting again.

    Note: Only do this once. After that the dough will become too tough and too dry.
11. Place the scones on a greased baking sheet.
12. Bake at 425°F (220°C, Gas Mark 7) for 12 to 15 minutes.

Serve warm

How To Make Strawberry Jam

Ingredients

2 pounds (900g) fresh strawberries, washed, dried, hulled and lightly chopped
4 cups (800g) white sugar
Juice of one lemon

Method

1. Put the strawberries, sugar and lemon juice in a large saucepan.
2. Over low heat, cook until all the sugar dissolves.
3. Turn up the heat to medium-high an bring to a full, rolling boil.
4. Boil rapidly, stirring frequently, for 15-20 minutes. The jam should be fairly thick.
5. Remove any froth from the top and remove saucepan from heat.
6. Pour into warm, sterile jam jars and allow to cool before sealing.
7. If jam is going to be used right away, refrigerate it after it has cooled. It will keep for about 2 weeks in the fridge.

If you want to keep it for longer, store in the freezer and thaw when needed.

Sterilize Jars

The easiest way to sterilize jam jars is to place them in your oven and bring the temperature up to 350°F (175°C, Gas Mark 4). Don't go any hotter as you may crack the glass. Put some newspaper on the shelf and lay the jars down so they don't touch each other.

Heat them for 20 minutes and use a good quality oven mitt to handle them.

Fill them while hot with the hot jam mixture.

You can also run your dishwasher on a rinse cycle timed to finish when your jam is ready. Only use this method if you have a sanitize setting on your dishwasher.

How To Make Clotted Cream

Clotted cream is a process. You start with unpasteurized cream and by slowly heating it, clots will form on the surface. It is easy to do but does take a long time. Is it worth it - absolutely.

Ingredients

4 cups (950 mL) unpasteurized whipping cream

The problem of course is that you cannot go to the grocery store and buy unpasteurized cream. So you have to make do with pasteurized cream. Avoid the ultra-pasteurized cream because it won't work.

Just buy whipping cream with the highest fat content you can find, probably 40%.

If you have happen to live in a dairy area and can persuade a local farmer to sell you unpasteurized cream then you are in for a real treat.

Method

1. Find an oven safe pot with a lid and pour in the cream. It should be a couple of inches deep but a little more or less is not critical.
2. Put the covered pot in the oven for 8 to 12 hours at 180°F (82°C)
3. The cream will form a think yellowish skin - that's the clotted cream.
4. Let the pot cool to room temperature then put it in the fridge for another 8 hours.
5. Scoop the cream off the top and put it in a serving dish. What's left in the pot is still good cream and can be used for baking.

SERVING

Traditionally the tea should be served with milk but if that's not the way you like it, don't do it. Homemade strawberry jam is always served with Devonshire Tea but if you have to buy it at least use a good quality preserve that has whole berries.

You can even buy scones at the bakers but there really isn't a substitute for the clotted cream. Don't let anyone tell you whipped cream is just as good because it's not the same at all.

Instant Pot Strawberry Jam

Making strawberry jam in your Instant Pot is a little easier than making it the traditional way. It requires less stirring and is less messy because it eliminates those inevitable splatters that occur when using a stovetop method.

Ingredients

2 pounds (900g) strawberries, cleaned, stemmed and roughly chopped
2½ cups (500g) granulated sugar
4 tablespoons (60 mL) lemon juice, preferably fresh

Method

1. Place all the ingredients in the Instant Pot and select the Sauté mode. Mix well and continue stirring until all the sugar has melted.
2. Turn off Sauté mode and place the lid on the Instant Pot. Turn the valve to "Sealing".
3. Select Manual mode and set for 6 minutes. When time is up, use a Natural Pressure Release.
4. Once the pressure is released, remove the lid and stir the jam.
5. If you want a less chunky jam, mash the strawberries using a potato masher. (optional)
6. Select the Sauté mode and allow the strawberries to cook for approximately 10 minutes. It should start to feel thicker.
7. Carefully spoon the jam into sterilized Mason jars while still warm and seal the jars "finger tight". Allow to cool on a wooden cutting board. The metal lids should seal as the jam cools. If any do not seal properly, use them first.

The jam should keep in the refrigerator for 2 to 3 months or in the freezer for 6 months.

Instant Pot Clotted Cream

Clotted cream is a must with Devonshire Tea but can be rather fiddly and time-consuming to make.

This Instant Pot recipe makes it much easier to achieve amazing results so that you can, indeed, have an authentic Devonshire Tea experience.

Ingredients

4 cups (950 mL) heavy cream (whipping cream) Note: DO NOT purchase ultra-pasteurized cream as it won't work.

Method

1. Pour the cream into Instant Pot insert and close lid and set the value to "Sealing".
2. Set Instant Pot mode to Yogurt Boil. To achieve this, press the Yogurt button and then the Adjust until you see the word "Boil".
3. When Instant Pot beeps, indicating that the boil setting is done, press the Keep Warm button. The Keep Warm mode maintains the temperature between 145°F and 172°F (63°C to 78°C).
4. Leave on the Keep Warm setting for 8 hours.
5. Turn off Instant Pot, remove the lid and remove insert. Place the insert on a wire rack to cool. Be careful not to agitate the cream too much. Agitating will cause the cream to mix back into the milk liquids underneath, reducing the amount of clotted cream you end up with.
6. Allow the cream to cool for about an hour at room temperature.
7. Cover the pot with plastic wrap and put in fridge for at least 8 hours, again, being careful not to agitate the cream.
8. After 8 to 12 hours the clotted cream will have thickened.
9. Using a slotted spoon, gently skim the thick layer of clotted cream from the surface, leaving the whey behind, and ladle into a jar or bowl. Sterilized Mason jars would work well.

This recipe will yield about 2 cups (480 mL), perhaps a little more, of clotted cream.

If you like your clotted cream to be a little less thick, stir some of the whey back into it.

DON'T throw the whey out! You can use it to make Whey Scones.

Refrigerate the clotted cream and use within 4-5 days.

Also refrigerate the whey and use it up within 4-5 days as well. You can substitute whey for buttermilk in any recipe that calls for buttermilk.

Whey Scones

After you've made your clotted cream, you won't want to waste the whey. This recipe makes lovely, fluffy scones and uses the leftover whey.

However, if you don't have any whey, you can always substitute buttermilk or regular whole milk.

Ingredients

> 2 cups (240g) all-purpose unbleached white flour
> 4 teaspoons (20 mL) baking powder
> 2 tablespoons (30g) cold butter
> 1 cup (250 mL) Whey

Method

1. Pre-heat the oven to 425°F (220°C, Gas Mark 7).
2. In a large bowl, combine the flour and baking powder. Mix well.
3. Using a pastry blender, or two knives, cut in the cold butter until the mixture resembles breadcrumbs or a coarse oatmeal.
4. Add the whey, mixing just enough to combine.
5. Turn the mixture out onto a lightly floured surface and gently knead to form a smooth dough.
6. With the palms of your hands, press the dough out to a thickness of about ½ inch (1.25 cm) overall.
7. Use a 2 to 2½ inch (5 to 6.3 cm) round cookie cutter to cut the scones out of the dough.
8. You can re-use any scraps left over from cutting the dough by reforming and cutting again. Note: Only do this once. After that the dough will become too tough and too dry.
9. Gently place the scones, close together but not touching, on a lightly greased baking sheet.
10. Brush each scone with a little whey (or milk).
11. Bake at 425°F (220°C, Gas Mark 7) for 12 to 15 minutes or until golden brown.
12. Remove from the oven and allow to cool on a wire rack.

Cornish Pasties

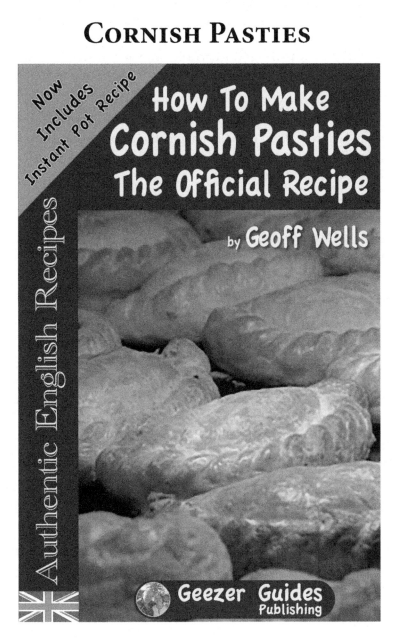

INTRODUCTION

Long before the card playing 4th Earl of Sandwich ordered his servants to bring him slices of meat between bread so he didn't have to interrupt his game, there was the pasty.

The first known references to pasties are from the thirteenth century, at the time of Henry III. Back then it was made mostly from venison and considered a luxury food item. Later it was adopted by the common man and made famous by the Cornish tin mines.

The recipe's thick pastry crust stayed warm for many hours and made a convenient, sturdy lunch for the miners to carry. One theory says that by handling them by the folded edge, which they discarded, they did not ingest the arsenic they got on their hands from mining tin.

Another folk tale says that the pastry must be sturdy enough to survive a drop down the mine shaft.

The Protected Pasty

In our present day world, the Cornish Pastry has Protected Geographical Indication (PGI) status in Europe. Which means by European law, to be called a "Cornish Pasty", this delectable pastry must have been made from a particular recipe and it must also have been made in Cornwall.

I can give you the official recipe but, unless you happen to live in Cornwall, you will just have to call it something else.

So, if you insist on calling it a Cornish Pastry and one day two burly tin miners with strange accents show up on your doorstep, all I can say is, "You were warned!"

Actually, even in Cornwall, you will find pasties with a variety of fillings. A pasty is actually defined by its familiar "D" shape rather than what is inside it. This is good because it allows me to include lots of pasty recipes that are still Authentic English Recipes.

Cornish Pasty Association

The Cornish Pasty Association has a web site where you can find the official recipe. This is what you see below but I translated from the original English so that it makes sense to North Americans.

I've also put a copy of a video all about Cornish Pasties on the Authentic English Recipes web site.

Lots Of Pasties

It can be fun to come up with original pasty filling combinations. Over the years I've tried lots of ideas, some of which have been total disasters and others that have become family favorites.

In this book you will find the pasty recipes that friends and family have voted the best.

The Official Cornish Pasty Recipe

SOURCE: http://www.cornishpastyassociation.co.uk/pasties.html

The Cornish Pasty Association, on their website, has this to say about a genuine Cornish Pasty -

A genuine Cornish pasty has a distinctive 'D' shape and is crimped on one side, never on top. The texture of the filling is chunky, made up of uncooked minced or roughly cut chunks of beef (not less than 12.5%), swede, potato, onion with a light seasoning. The pastry casing is golden in colour, savoury, glazed with milk or egg and robust enough to retain its shape throughout the cooking and cooling process without splitting or cracking. The pasty is slow-baked and no artificial flavourings or additives must be used. And, perhaps most importantly, it must also be made in Cornwall.

Ingredients

SERVINGS: 4

Pastry

500 grams strong bread flour *(It is important to use a stronger flour than normal as you need the extra strength in the gluten to produce strong pliable pastry.)*
120 grams white shortening
25 grams cake margarine
5 grams Salt
175 grams cold water

Filling

450 grams beef skirt
450 grams potato
250 grams swede
200 grams Onion
Salt & Pepper, 2/1 Ratio
Clotted Cream, Optional
Butter, Optional

Method

Pastry

1. Mix fat lightly into flour until it resembles breadcrumbs.
2. Add water and beat in a food mixer until pastry clears and becomes elastic. This will take longer than normal pastry but it gives the pastry the strength that is needed to hold the filling and retain a good shape.
3. Leave to rest for 3 hours in a refrigerator, this is a very important stage as it is almost impossible to roll and shape the pastry when fresh.

Filling

Chop the above finely then add to the rolled out circles of pastry raw. Layer the vegetables and meat adding plenty of seasoning. Put a dollop of cream or a knob of butter on top. Then bring the pastry around and crimp together. Try practicing on a potato first or just flatten like a turnover and mark with a fork. Crimping is the secret to a true Cornish pasty but it really has to be taught it is almost impossible to describe.

Cooking time and temperature

Gas No 6 approximately 50 minutes - 1 hour

Electric 210 approximately 50 minutes -1 hour

Fan assisted 165 approximately 40 minutes

The Official Cornish Pasty ~ US Version

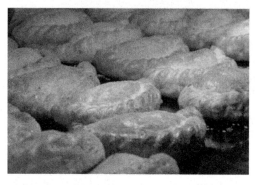

Translated from the original English

If you found the original version a little hard to follow here is the translation, plus a few notes for those of you that don't do a lot of baking.

I didn't just rely on some conversion program to make the ingredient list US friendly, I actually measured everything - then enjoyed the results.

INGREDIENTS

SHORT CRUST PASTRY

    4 cups flour (I used All Purpose which worked just fine, but use bread flour if you have it.)
    ¼ pound (4 oz.) lard (you can use vegetable shortening but lard is better.)
    2 teaspoon margarine (Use the bricks rather than tub margarine as it is firmer.)
    1 teaspoon salt
    ¾ cup cold water

FILLING

    1 pound beef skirt (skirt or flank may be difficult to find, substitute good steak like sirloin.)
    3½ cups potato (thinly sliced, roughly chopped)
    2½ cups rutabaga (thinly sliced, roughly chopped)
    2 cups onion (thinly sliced, roughly chopped)
    salt & pepper, 2/1 ratio
    clotted cream, optional
    butter, optional

Method

Pastry

1. Cut the fat into the flour until it resembles bread crumbs.
2. Add water and beat with a food mixer until the pastry clears and becomes elastic. This will take longer than normal pastry but it gives the pastry the strength that is needed to hold the filling and retain a good shape.
3. Leave it to rest for 3 hours in a refrigerator, this is a very important stage as it is almost impossible to roll and shape the pastry when it is fresh.

Filling

1. Remove any fat or skin from the meat then cut into thin (¼ inch) strips about 1 inch long. Divide into four piles.
2. Roughly chop the potato, rutabaga and onion. You want thin slices that will cook easily and not fall out of the pasty when you eat it.
3. Divide the pastry into four equal balls then roll each ball out to a thickness of about 1/8 inch and cut 4 circles the size of a dinner plate - 9 inches to 10 inches in diameter.
4. Divide each vegetable into four piles then layer the potato, rutabaga, onion and meat across the diameter of each pastry circle. Shake a generous portion of pepper and salt over each pile. Put a pat of butter on top of each filling pile.
5. Fold the pastry over the filling and crimp the edge. Crimping is a squeeze and twist motion that is easy once you know how. To see how the experts do it see this crimping guide.

http://www.cornishpastyassociation.co.uk/about-the-pasty/make-your-own-genuine-cornish-pasty/

6. Put the four pasties on a baking sheet and brush them with an egg wash made from one beaten egg and 1 tablespoon of water.
7. Put the baking sheet on the center rack of a pre-heated 400°F oven. After 30 minutes brush again with the egg wash. Cook for a total of 50 - 60 minutes, or until the pasties are golden brown.
8. Serve as a complete meal with a light salad on the side.

Serves: 4

You Might Want More Meat

That was the translation of the official recipe but we find it a little light on meat and the overall serving size a little too big. I suggest you double the quantity of meat to 2 pounds and increase the servings to six.

Flaky Pastry Recipe

If you prefer a lighter, flakier pastry this recipe will produce perfect pastry every time. I'm just including the basic recipe but if you want a complete pastry making course take a look at my wife's book, "[How To Make Perfect Pastry Every Time](https://ebooks.geezerguides.com/make-perfect-pastry-every-time/)"

Note: This pastry will not survive a fall down a mine shaft.

Ingredients

5½ cups (660g) all purpose flour
2 teaspoons (10 mL) salt
1 pound (450g) lard
1 large egg
1 tablespoon (15 mL) white vinegar
water

Method

1. Measure out 5 cups (600g) of flour, keeping ½ cup (60g) in reserve.
2. Add the salt to the flour and mix well.
3. Use a pastry blender to cut the lard into the flour and salt mixture. Blend until the mixture resembles coarse oatmeal.
4. In a separate liquid measuring cup, break the egg into the cup and beat slightly. Add the tablespoon of vinegar and then just enough water to bring the measurement up to one cup (240 mL).
5. Mix the liquid into the flour mixture. Initially, use a fork to mix in the liquid, then get in there with your hands to complete the mixing.
6. You don't want to over-mix, but you want a smooth dough that's not very sticky. It should pull away from your fingers easily. Add a bit more flour if you need to, but not too much as you'll be adding more flour when you roll out the dough.
7. Cover the dough with plastic wrap and chill for about an hour. Dough rolls out better when it's cold.

    Hint: It's a good idea to chill the rolling pin as well.

8. Once the dough has chilled, take about 1/6th of the dough and make it into a thick, flat circle. Place it on a lightly floured surface and roll it out. You may need to dust with more flour so the dough doesn't stick to the rolling pin or the rolling surface.
9. Cut into desired shapes for whatever recipe you are using.

Unofficial Cornish Pasty Appetizers

For appetizers we change the recipe around a little bit because of the smaller size. Mainly, we pre-cook the filling because the bite-size pasties are not in the oven long enough to cook the meat. We also use hamburger, onions and carrots plus some seasoning for the filling.

You can use either the flaky pastry recipe above or the original short crust pastry, but I would recommend the flaky. Since these are bite size you will be cutting much smaller pastry circles. About 4½ inches is a good size. That is the size of the plastic lids that come with containers of yogurt, sour cream, cottage cheese, etc.

This is actually the Cornish pasty recipe I grew up with except that my mother made them full size. The poultry seasoning is not a misprint, that's what my mother called "spice". She used a very limited palette of spices but the taste just works - try it, you'll like it.

Ingredients

1 pound (450g) lean ground beef
1 carrot, finely diced
1 medium potato, finely diced
1 medium onion, finely diced
2 cubes beef bouillon, or 1 tablespoon (15 mL) liquid Bovril™
1 tablespoon (15 mL) poultry seasoning
2 cups (480 mL) warm water
1½ tablespoons (22 mL) cornstarch
pastry dough, enough for a 2 crust pie

Method

1. In a large saucepan, over medium-high heat, brown the ground beef until it is no longer pink. Be sure to break up the ground beef so there are no large lumps.
2. Remove from heat and drain off the fat.
3. To the browned ground beef, add the finely diced carrots, onions and potatoes and mix thoroughly.
4. Add the 2 cups (480 mL) of warm water to the saucepan then crumble the beef bouillon cube into the beef and water.
5. Mix the cornstarch with just enough water to create a thin paste. Set aside.
6. Return the saucepan to the stove and heat over medium-high heat until the mixture begins to boil. Make sure that the bouillon cubes have completely dissolved. If you can get liquid Bovril™, that is the better choice.
7. Reduce heat slightly and allow mixture to simmer for about 5 - 8 minutes to ensure the vegetables get cooked properly.

8. With the meat mixture still simmering, stir the cornstarch mixture to make sure there are no lumps and gradually add it to the simmering meat mixture, stirring constantly.
9. Once the mixture is thickened (it must be very thick and not runny at all), remove from heat and cool completely. If you try to add a hot mixture to the pastry, the pastry will break down and it just won't work.

PRE-HEAT THE OVEN

10. Before you start to assemble the appetizer-size Cornish pasties, turn on your oven so that it will be at 400°F (200°C, Gas Mark 6). when you're ready to bake them.

PREPARING THE PASTRY

11. Roll the pastry out to about 1/8" (.3 cm) thick and then cut circles about 4½ inches (11.5 cm) in diameter (often the lid of a small, plastic margarine container is about the right size - just press it into the dough to create the circle).

FILLING THE PASTRY

12. Before you fill the pastry, wet the edges of the circle. This will help to seal the pastry.
13. Place about 2 tablespoons of the filling in the middle of the circle of pastry.
14. GENTLY, fold the pastry over like you would for a turnover, and press all along the edge to seal.
15. GENTLY transfer each pasty to a slightly greased baking sheet.
16. The number you end up with will be determined by either the amount filling you use and the amount of pastry you have. Either leftover pastry or filling can be frozen for use later.
17. Baking the Baby Cornish Pasties
18. Bake at 400°F (200°C, Gas Mark 6) for 15 - 20 minutes. You want to pastry to be golden brown. The filling may bubble out a little, but that's okay, just as long as the pasty isn't coming apart altogether.
19. When the pastry is golden brown, remove from the oven and cool on a wire rack.

These pasty appetizers can be served hot, warm or room temperature.

Savory Pasties

If you have run out of ideas for different lunch time sandwiches try taking one of these to the office. Microwaves are not good for pastry but if you're careful you can warm them up without making them soggy.

- ❖ Vegetarian Pasty
- ❖ Cheese, Mushroom and Leek
- ❖ Ham, Swiss Cheese and Asparagus
- ❖ Sausage Pasty
- ❖ Pizza Pasty
- ❖ Asian Pasty
- ❖ Jerk Chicken Pasty

Vegetarian Pasty

We are not vegetarians but sometimes we enjoy a meatless meal. This is a nice flavourful combination you can try for a change or to serve to your vegetarian friends. To be truly vegetarian you will have to substitute vegetable shortening for the lard in the flaky pastry recipe.

Ingredients

>   pastry dough
>   ½ cup (75g) onion, diced
>   ½ cup (115g) cabbage, shredded
>   ¼ cup (15g) carrot, diced
>   ½ cup (115g) potato, diced
>   ½ cup (40g) mushrooms, sliced
>   2 tablespoons (30 mL) vegetable oil
>   1 teaspoon (5 mL) sea salt, freshly ground
>   ½ teaspoon (2.5 mL) black pepper, freshly ground
>   1 tablespoon (15 mL) balsamic vinegar

Method

1. In a large bowl, combine all ingredients, except the pastry, and toss until well mixed.
2. Refrigerate for at least one hour, preferably overnight, to allow flavor to combine and to allow the vinegar to begin to soften the veggies.
3. Remove the mixture from the fridge and let it warm up to room temperature before filling the pastry.
4. Pre-heat the oven to 400°F (200°C, Gas Mark 6)
5. Place filled pasties on a lightly greased baking sheet and bake for 15 - 25 minutes depending on the size of pasty you have chosen to make. The pastry should be golden brown.
6. Remove from the oven and allow to cool on a wire rack for a few minutes, then serve.

Serves: 2

Cheese, Mushroom and Leek

Here is another filling combination that might be classified as vegetarian depending on how you feel about cheese. You might also need to substitute vegetable shortening for the lard in the <u>pastry</u>.

Ingredients

   pastry dough, enough for a 2 crust pie
   6 ounces (170g) old cheddar cheese
   2 portobello mushrooms
   2 leeks, thinly sliced
   butter
   sea salt, to taste
   black pepper, to taste

Method

1. Pre-heat the oven to 400°F (200°C, Gas Mark 6)
2. Roll out the pastry dough and cut out four 8 inch circles.
3. Clean the portobello mushrooms and remove the stems and gills. The slice each mushroom into 6 slices.
4. Cut the cheddar cheese into 4 equal strips about 5 - 6 inches long and about ½ inch thick on each side.
5. On each pastry circle arrange the cheddar cheese, 3 slices of the Portobelo mushroom, half of a thinly sliced leek (white part only). Put a small pat of butter on top and then salt and pepper to taste.
6. Wet the edges of the pastry and carefully fold the pastry over the filling. Seal by pressing the edges together and bake at 400°F (200°C, Gas Mark 6) for 15 - 20 minutes or until the pastry is golden brown.
7. Remove from oven and cool on a wire rack. Let cool for about 5 minutes and serve.

Serves: 4

Ham, Swiss Cheese and Asparagus

This makes a tasty, different lunch and it is good hot or cold. Try taking some on your next picnic.

Ingredients

   pastry dough, enough for a 2 crust pie
   8 ounces (225g) Black Forest Ham, 2 thick slices
   4 ounces (110g) Swiss cheese, sliced
   12 spears asparagus, washed and trimmed
   butter
   sea salt, to taste
   black pepper, to taste

Method

1. Pre-heat oven to 400°F (200°C, Gas Mark 6)
2. Roll out the pastry and cut out four 8 inch circles.
3. One each pastry circle arrange 2 ounces of Black Forest ham, 1 ounce of Swiss Cheese and three asparagus spears (cut the spears to fit within the pastry, if necessary). Place a small pat of butter on top and salt and pepper to taste.
4. Wet the edges of the pastry and gently fold over filling. Seal the edges of the pastry.
5. Transfer pasties to slightly greased backing sheet and bake at 400°F (200°C, Gas Mark 6) for 15-20 minutes or until pastry is golden brown.
6. Remove from oven and allow to cool slightly on a wire rack.

Serves: 4

Sausage Pasty

For a tasty variation add a thinly sliced apple Add the raw apple just before you seal the pasty and bake.

Ingredients

    pastry dough, enough for a 2 crust pie
    12 ounces (340g) sausage meat
    ½ cup (75g) onion, diced
    ½ cup (115g) potato, diced
    1 cube beef bouillon
    ½ cup (120 mL) water
    1 tablespoon (15 mL) cornstarch

Method

1. In a medium skillet, brown the sausage meat until it is no longer pink. Drain the sausage meat and set aside.
2. In the same skillet, brown the onions and the potatoes slightly - about 3 minutes - and return the drained sausage meat to the skillet.
3. Add the ½ cup (120 mL) water and crumbled bouillon cube to the skillet and bring to a boil. Meanwhile, in a small dish, mix the cornstarch with just enough water to make a thin paste.
4. Once the sausage mixture has come to a boil, reduce the heat and simmer the mixture for a minute or two. Then, while it is still simmering, gradually stir in the cornstarch mixture and allow the meat mixture to simmer until it has thickened well.
5. Remove from heat and allow to cool to room temperature before filling the pastry.
6. Pre-heat the oven to 400°F (200°C, Gas Mark 6)
7. Roll out the pastry and cut out four 8 inch (20 cm) circles.
8. Fill each pastry circle with ¼ of the sausage mixture. Wet the edges on the pastry and carefully fold the pastry over the filling. Seal the edges of the pastry.
9. Place pasties on a slightly greased baking sheet and bake at 400°F (200°C, Gas Mark 6) for 15 - 20 minutes or until pastry is golden brown.
10. Remove from the oven and cool on a wire rack.

Serves: 4

Pizza Pasty

Make a batch or two and refrigerate before the big game. When the gang comes over just warm them for 10 minutes at 300°F. Something a little different in the way of finger food.

Ingredients

    pastry dough, enough for a 2 crust pie
    4 ounces (110g) pepperoni, sliced
    2 ounces (55g) mozzarella cheese, shredded
    ¼ cup (40g) onion, finely chopped
    ¼ cup (60g) green bell pepper, finely chopped
    ½ cup (120 mL) pasta sauce

Method

1. Pre-heat oven to 375°F (190°C, Gas Mark 5)
2. Roll out the pastry and cut out four 8 inch (20 cm) circles.
3. On each pastry circle place 1 ounce (27.5g) of sliced pepperoni, 1 tablespoon (15 mL) of chopped onion, 1 tablespoon (15 mL) of chopped green pepper and ¼ of the shredded mozzarella. Top with 2 tablespoons (30 mL) of pasta sauce.
4. Wet the edges of the pastry and carefully fold over the filling and seal the edges.
5. Place on a lightly greased baking sheet and bake at 375°F (190°C, Gas Mark 5) for 15 - 20 minutes or until pastry is golden brown.
6. Remove from oven and cool on a wire rack. Allow them to cool for several minutes as the sauce and cheese will be very hot right out of the oven.

Serves: 4

Asian Pasty

Make this a little different by serving an orange sauce beside the pasty.

Ingredients

    pastry dough, enough for a 2 crust pie
    ½ cup (50g) bean sprouts
    ½ cup (70g) water chestnuts, coarsely chopped
    ½ cup (40g) mushrooms, sliced
    ½ cup (65g) cooked chicken, coarsely chopped
    ¼ cup (60 mL) soy sauce
    2 tablespoons (25g) sugar

Method

1. In a large bowl, combine the bean sprouts, water chestnuts, cooked chicken, soy sauce and sugar. Mix well and refrigerate for about one hour.
2. Once the chicken mixture has chilled for an hour, pre-heat oven to 400°F (200°C, Gas Mark 6).
3. Roll out the pastry and cut into four 8 inch (20 cm) circles.
4. On each pastry circle place ¼ of the chicken mixture.
5. Wet the edges of the pastry and carefully fold over the filling. Seal the edges of the pastry.
6. Transfer each pasty to a slightly greased baking sheet and bake at 400°F (200°C, Gas Mark 6) for 15 - 20 minutes or until the pastry is golden brown.
7. Remove from oven and cool slightly on a wire rack.

Sauce Ingredients

    1 - 11 ounce (300g) can mandarin oranges
    2 teaspoons (10 mL) cornstarch

Sauce Method

Drain the oranges and thicken the juice with the cornstarch. To do that just heat the juice in a small thick bottom saucepan. Mix the cornstarch with just enough water to make it pourable. When the juice is almost boiling add the cornstarch while stirring the juice rapidly. Remove from heat and fold in the orange segments.

Serves: 4

Jerk Chicken Pasty

The 2 tablespoons (30 mL) of Jerk seasoning is just a suggestion and I expect you to vary the amount depending on how hot you like it. Consider serving a side dish of sliced cucumber, tomato, and sour cream.

Ingredients

pastry dough, enough for a 2 crust pie
1 pound (450g) boneless chicken breast, cubed
1 tablespoon (15 mL) butter, melted
2 tablespoons (30 mL) Jerk seasoning
1 egg yolk
1 tablespoon (15 mL) water

Method

1. In a large glass bowl, combine the chicken and melted butter and toss until well coated.
2. Note: The chicken should be diced fairly small so that it will cook through.
3. Sprinkle the chicken mixture with the Jerk seasoning and toss until the chicken is well coated. Cover and refrigerate for at least one hour.

    Note: Jerk seasoning is available in most grocery stores.

4. When the chicken mixture has been chilled for at least an hour, pre-heat the oven to 375°F (190°C, Gas Mark 5).
5. Roll out the pastry dough and cut into four 8 inch (20 cm) circles.
6. On each pastry circle, place ¼ of the chicken mixture. Wet the edges of the pastry and carefully fold the pastry over the filling and seal the edges.
7. Transfer the pasties to a lightly greased baking sheet.
8. In a small bowl, whisk together the egg yolk and water. Using a pastry brush, brush the tops of each pasty with the egg yolk mixture.
9. Bake the pasties at 375°F (190°C, Gas Mark 5) for 20 - 15 minutes or until the pastry is golden brown.
10. Remove from oven and allow to cool slightly on a wire rack.

Serves: 4

Dessert Pasties

A light entrée paired with a dessert pasty can make an interesting switch from the usual meal plan. For a really decadent treat add clotted, whipped or ice cream to any of the dessert pasties.

- ❖ Peach & Walnut Pasty
- ❖ Bumbleberry Pasties
- ❖ Banana & Chocolate Pasty
- ❖ Banana Split Pasty
- ❖ Apple and Walnut Pasty

Peach & Walnut Pasty

Walnuts are a very soft nut so you get the surprising taste without having to crunch through what you may think was a mistake by the cook.

Ingredients

>   pastry dough, enough for a 2 crust pie
>   2 peaches, peeled, stoned and sliced
>   ¼ cup (30g) walnut pieces
>   2 tablespoons (15g) all purpose flour
>   ¼ cup (45g) brown sugar
>   butter

Method

1. Pre-heat oven to 400°F (200°C, Gas Mark 6).
2. Cut each peach into eight slices.
3. Note: You can use canned, sliced peaches, just be sure to drain them well. You can always use the juice to make a sauce later.
4. Roll out the pastry and cut out four 8 inch (20 cm) circles.
5. On each pastry circle, arrange 4 peach slices and 1 tablespoon (7.5g) of walnut pieces. Sprinkle with ½ tablespoon (3.75g) of flour and then 1 tablespoon (11g) of brown sugar and then put a small pat of butter on top.
6. Wet the edges of the pastry. Then carefully fold the pastry over the filling and seal the edges.
7. Transfer the pasties to a lightly greased baking sheet and bake at 400°F (200°C, Gas Mark 6) for 10 - 15 minutes or until pastry is golden brown.
8. Remove from oven and cool on a wire rack.

Serves: 4

Bumbleberry Pasties

Go ahead and substitute any fresh summer berries that are in season, Gooseberries, strawberries, red and black currents are all good choices.

Instead of ice cream try some Bird's Custard on your warm bumbleberry pasty. It goes particularly well with this and the banana chocolate. You'll find it in any UK or Canadian supermarket. If you're in the US you may find it but your best bet is our website

https://ebooks.geezerguides.com/products-from-our-books/

Ingredients

pastry dough, enough for a 2 crust pie
¼ cup (30g) raspberries
¼ cup (25g) blueberries
¼ cup (25g) blackberries
¼ cup (25g) cranberries, fresh or frozen
¼ cup (50g) sugar
¼ cup (30g) all purpose flour

Method

1. Wash all the fruit well and drain any excess water.
2. In a large bowl, mix together all the fruit, sugar and flour. Toss well to make sure all the fruit is well coated with the sugar and the flour.
3. Pre-heat oven to 400°F (200°C, Gas Mark 6).
4. Roll out the pastry and cut into four 8 inch (20 cm) circles.
5. Fill each pastry circle with ¼ of the fruit mix. Wet the edges of the pastry, then carefully fold the pastry over the filling and seal the edges.
6. Place the pasties on a lightly greased cooking sheet and bake at 400°F (200°C, Gas Mark 6) for 10 - 15 minutes or until the pastry is golden brown.
7. Remove from oven and cool on a wire rack.

Serves: 4

Banana & Chocolate Pasty

Just because the recipe says semi-sweet chocolate chips doesn't mean you can't substitute a Cadbury Flake™. I only put the chocolate chips in because that's what you can easily find in any US grocery store. If you want the real thing check out our web site.

https://ebooks.geezerguides.com/products-from-our-books/

Ingredients

    pastry dough, enough for 1 pie crust
    2 bananas
    6 tablespoons (65g) semi-sweet chocolate chips
    5 teaspoons (20g) sugar

Method

1. Pre-heat oven to 400°F (200°C, Gas Mark 6).
2. Roll out the pastry and cut out four 8 inch (20 cm) circles.
3. Cut each banana in half and place one half on each pastry round.
4. Sprinkle one teaspoon (5g) of sugar over each banana half.
5. Sprinkle 1½ tablespoons (16g) of chocolate chips over each banana half.
6. Wet the edges of the pastry, fold over the filling and seal.
7. With a pastry brush, brush a little water on top of each pasty and sprinkle some sugar on the top.
8. Place each pasty on a slightly greased baking sheet.
9. Bake at 400°F (200°C, Gas Mark 6) for 10 - 15 minutes or until pastry is golden brown.
10. Remove from oven and cool on a wire rack. Allow to cool for at least 5 minutes.
11. Serve with a scoop of ice cream on the side, or just have as is.
12. You can also allow them to cool completely. That way the chocolate will solidify again.

Serves: 4

Banana Split Pasty

The flaky pastry is good hot, warm or cold so this delicious dessert can be served any way you want. Try it with afternoon tea for a quick energy boost to get you through the rest of the work day.

Ingredients

   pastry dough, enough for a 2 crust pie
   1 large banana
   4 strawberries, sliced
   ½ cup (100g) pineapple chunks, well drained
   ¼ cup (45g) chocolate chips
   4 scoops vanilla ice cream

Method

1. Pre-heat oven to 400°F (200°C, Gas Mark 6).
2. Roll out pastry dough and cut into four 8 inch (20 cm) circles.
3. Slice the banana lengthwise and then in half.
4. On each pastry circle, place one banana quarter then top with 1 sliced strawberry, ¼ of the pineapple chunks and 1 tablespoon of chocolate chips.
5. Wet the edges of the pastry. Then, carefully fold the pastry over the filling and seal the edges.
6. Place the pasties on a lightly greased baking sheet and bake at 400°F (200°C, Gas Mark 6) for 10 - 15 minutes, or until the pastry is golden brown.
7. Remove from oven and cool on a wire rack.
8. To continue the banana split theme, serve with a scoop of vanilla ice cream.

Serves: 4

Apple and Walnut Pasty

If you are a little more adventurous substitute ¼ cup of chopped figs for the walnuts, then top with a generous helping of Bird's Custard.

Ingredients

>   pastry dough, enough for a 2 crust pie
>   2 baking apples, washed, peeled, cored and sliced
>   ¼ cup (30g) walnut pieces
>   ¼ cup (45g) brown sugar
>   2 tablespoons (15g) all purpose flour
>   1 teaspoon (5 mL) cinnamon
>   ¼ teaspoon (1.25 mL) black pepper
>   butter

Method

1. Pre-heat oven to 400°F (200°C, Gas Mark 6).
2. In a large bowl, toss together the apple slices, walnut pieces, brown sugar, flour, cinnamon and pepper. Make sure the apple slices and walnut pieces get well coated.
3. Roll out the pastry dough and cut into four 8 inch (20 cm) circles.
4. Place ¼ of the apple mixture on each pastry circle. Place a small pat of butter on top of the filling. Wet the edges of the pastry and gently fold the pastry over the filling. Seal the edges of the pastry.
5. Transfer the pasties to a lightly greased baking sheet and bake at 400°F (200°C, Gas Mark 6) for 10 - 15 minutes or until pastry is golden brown.
6. Remove from oven and cool on a wire rack.

Serves: 4

~~~~

Instant Pot Cornish Pasty Appetizers Filling

This recipe only explains how to cook the filling in your Instant Pot.

Because of the size of these appetizers, the filling needs to be pre-cooked because they won't be in the oven long enough for the filling to cook thoroughly.

To make the appetizers, once the filling is cooked and cooled, please refer to the regular recipe on page 10.

Ingredients

- 1 pound (450g) lean ground beef
- 1 tablespoon (15 mL) poultry seasoning
- 1 carrot, finely diced
- 1 medium potato, finely diced
- 1 medium onion, finely diced
- 2 cups (480 mL) beef broth
- 1½ tablespoons (22 mL) cornstarch

Method

1. Using the Instant Pot Sauté mode, brown the ground beef until it is no loner pink. Be sure to break up the ground beef so there are no large lumps.
2. Turn off the Sauté mode and drain off any excess fat.
3. To the browned ground beef, add the poultry seasoning, finely diced carrots, onions and potatoes and mix thoroughly.
4. Add the 2 cups (480 mL) of beef broth and stir well.
5. Put the lid on the Instant Pot and lock it. Make sure the valve is in the "Sealing" position.
6. Select the Manual setting and set cooking time for 5 minutes.
7. Once the cooking time is completed, do a Quick Release.
8. While you're waiting for the pressure to release completely, in a small dish, mix the cornstarch with just enough water to create a thin paste.
9. Once the pressure has released, remove the Instant Pot lid and select Sauté mode. Bring the filling mixture to a simmer and slowly drizzle in the cornstarch and water mixture. Stir constantly as mixture thickens (it must be very thick and not runny at all).
10. Turn off the Instant Pot, remove the inner pot and set it aside so the filling mixture can cool to room temperature.
11. The filling needs to be cooled because if you try to add a hot mixture to the pastry, the pastry will break down and it just won't work.
12. Follow the instructions on how to create and bake the Cornish Pasty Appetizers.

BRITISH CAKES

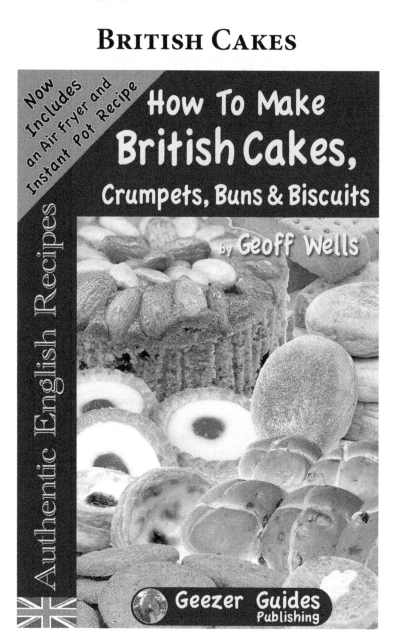

INTRODUCTION

Most of the books in this series are more about the method and ingredients of the recipes rather than exact quantities. This one is a little different as it is all about baking and baking just won't work unless you get the chemistry right.

These are my mother's recipes, modified for the North American measuring system. I have also changed any reference to self-raising flour because it is not widely available here.

I also want to thank my wife Vicky for developing the bread machine versions which will help to make these classic British favorites easier to make and therefore more available to busy cooks.

Bakewell Tarts

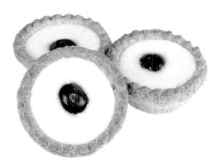

Bakewell tarts were one of my favorite treats growing up. The hard icing and the taste of the almond with the raspberry jam are sure to make these as popular in your family as they are in mine.

Ingredients

24 unbaked tart shells
Filling
½ cup (115g) butter
⅓ cup (80 mL) almond paste
½ cup (100g) sugar
3 eggs, slightly beaten
⅓ cup (40g) all purpose flour
1 cup (240 mL) raspberry jam

Icing

1 ⅓ cups (135g) confectioners sugar
2 tablespoons (30 mL) milk

Garnish

12 maraschino cherries, halved

Method

Pre-heat the oven to 400°F (200°C, Gas Mark 6).

In a medium bowl, beat the butter with an electric mixer on low until creamy. Gradually add the almond paste and sugar and continue to beat on low speed until smooth. Add the eggs one at a time while continuing to beat on low speed. Fold in the flour just until it is well blended.

Spoon a heaping teaspoon of jam into each tart shell. Then spoon the filling into each shell, dividing it equally between all of the shells.

Bake the tarts in a 400°F (200°C, Gas Mark 6) oven for about 12 to 15 minutes, or until they are golden brown.

Remove from the oven and cool completely on a wire rack.

TO MAKE THE ICING

In a small bowl combine the confectioners sugar (icing sugar) with about 2 tablespoons of water and stir until smooth. Spoon the icing over the completely cooled tarts.

To garnish, place a maraschino cherry half in the middle of each tart and press slightly into the icing. Allow the icing to hardened slightly before serving.

Servings: 24

English Shortbread

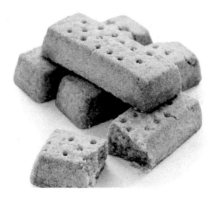

Store bought shortbread always seems so expensive for something so simple to make. Also by making it yourself you know it won't come with unwanted chemicals.

Ingredients

> 1 cup (225g) salted butter, DO NOT SUBSTITUTE MARGARINE
> ½ cup (100g) sugar
> 3 cups (360g) all purpose flour

Method

Pre-heat the oven to 375°F (190°C, Gas Mark 5).

Cream the butter and sugar together until light and fluffy.

Gradually mix in the flour using a fork and then your hands. The mixture may be a bit crumbly.

Firmly and evenly press the mixture into a 9 inch by 13 inch (23 cm x 33 cm) greased baking pan.

With a fork, prick the dough well, then lightly score the dough, with a very sharp knife, into bars.

Bake at 375°F (190°C, Gas Mark 5) for about 20 minutes or until it is a light golden brown.

Remove the shortbread from the oven and allow to cool completely on a wire rack.

When the shortbread has cooled completely, cut it into bars along the score lines.

Servings: 12

SCONES

Serve these scones instead of bread for a delicious change of pace.

INGREDIENTS

2 cups (240g) all purpose flour
3 teaspoons (15 mL) baking powder
½ teaspoon (2.5 mL) salt
2 tablespoons (25g) sugar
⅓ cup (75g) shortening
2 large eggs, slightly beaten
½ cup (120 mL) whole milk or cream, approximately

METHOD

Pre-heat the oven to 425°F (220°C, Gas Mark 7).

In a large bowl, combine the flour, baking powder, salt and sugar. Mix well.

Cut in the shortening with a pastry blender until the mixture resembles a coarse corn meal.

In a separate measuring cup, add enough milk to the slightly beaten eggs to make ¾ cup (180 mL). Mix well.

While stirring with a fork, add just enough of the liquid to make a soft dough. Continue stirring until all of the flour disappears.

On a lightly floured surface, knead the dough for about 30 seconds.

Either pat the dough down, or roll it out, to about ½ inch (1.25 cm) thick.

Cut into rounds with a cookie cutter. You should get 10 to 12 scones.

You can re-use any scrap left over from cutting the dough by reforming and cutting again.

Note: Only do this once. After that the dough will become too tough and too dry.
Place the scones on a greased baking sheet and bake at 425°F (220°C, Gas Mark 7) for 12 to 15 minutes.

Serve warm.

Servings: 12

Chelsea Buns

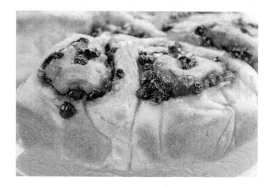

Chelsea buns look very much like cinnamon buns but the dough is very different. Chelsea buns are made with yeast and are like a sweet bread.

Ingredients

    1 cup (240 mL) milk, room temperature
    1 teaspoon (5 mL) salt
    2 eggs, room temperature
    2 tablespoons (30g) butter, softened
    3 cups (360g) all purpose flour
    1½ teaspoons (7.5 mL) yeast
    1½ cups (180g) dried mixed fruit, finely chopped
    ½ cup (90g) light brown sugar
    ½ teaspoon (2.5 mL) ground cinnamon
    ⅛ teaspoon (1.25 mL) ground nutmeg
    ⅛ teaspoon (1.25 mL) ground ginger
    ⅛ teaspoon (1.25 mL) ground allspice
    ⅛ teaspoon (1.25 mL) ground cloves
    ¼ cup (55g) butter, melted

Glaze

    ¼ cup (25g) superfine sugar
    ¼ cup (60 mL) milk

Method

Combine the flour and the salt in a large bowl. Create a depression in the middle of the flour and add the dried yeast.

In a small saucepan, heat the milk and butter together over medium heat until the butter melts and the mixture is lukewarm.

Add the milk mixture and the eggs to the flour mixture and stir until the mixture forms a soft dough.

Turn the dough out onto a well floured work surface and knead for about five minutes. Add more flour, if necessary, until the dough is smooth, elastic and no longer sticks to your hands.

Lightly oil a large bowl. Place the dough in the bowl and turn it so that the dough gets a light covering of oil. Cover the bowl with plastic wrap and let it stand in a warm area for about an hour. The dough should double in size.

Note: the best place for the dough to rise is in the oven with only the oven light turned on.

Punch down the dough and roll it out on a lightly floured surface to form a rectangle approximately 9 inches (23 cm) by 22 inches (55 cm). Mix together the dried fruit, brown sugar and spices. Brush the dough with the melted butter and sprinkle with the fruit mixture. Roll up the dough, from the long side, into a Swiss roll shape and cut into 18 equal pieces using a very sharp knife.

Arrange the buns, cut side down, in a lightly buttered 9 inch by 13 inch (23 cm x 33 cm) baking pan. Lightly brush the tops of the buns with melted butter and cover with plastic wrap. Allow the buns to rise in a warm area for about 30-45 minutes. The buns should be touching each other and the dough will be springy.

Note: the ideal place for the buns to rise is in the oven with just the oven light on.
Before pre-heating the oven, remove the risen buns and, carefully, remove the plastic wrap. Then, pre-heat the oven to 375°F (190°C, Gas Mark 5).

Bake at 375°F (190°C, Gas Mark 5) for about 20 minutes, until the buns are golden brown and cooked through.

Remove from the oven and cool on a wire rack for about 10 minutes, then drizzle with the sugar glaze.

To make the glaze

In a small saucepan heat the milk and sugar oven medium heat, stirring constantly with a wooden spoon, until the sugar dissolves and it comes to a slight boil. Reduce the heat to low and simmer for 2-3 minutes.

Note: be sure to watch this carefully as it can boil over or burn very easily.
To serve, gently pull the Chelsea buns apart. They can be served warm or cold. They also freeze well.

Servings: 18

Chelsea Buns
(Bread Machine Method)

The ingredients are the same but if you use a bread machine the job of mixing the dough is a lot easier.

Ingredients

   1 cup (240 mL) milk, room temperature
   1 teaspoon (5 mL) salt
   2 eggs, room temperature
   2 tablespoons (30g) butter, softened
   3 cups (360g) all purpose flour
   1½ teaspoons (7.5 mL) yeast
   1½ cups (180g) dried mixed fruit, finely chopped
   ½ cup (90g) light brown sugar
   ½ teaspoon (2.5 mL) ground cinnamon
   ⅛ teaspoon (1.25 mL) ground nutmeg
   ⅛ teaspoon (1.25 mL ground ginger
   ⅛ teaspoon (1.25 mL) ground allspice
   ⅛ teaspoon (1.25 mL) ground cloves
   ¼ cup (55g) butter, melted

Glaze

   ¼ cup (25g) superfine sugar
   ¼ cup (60 mL) milk

Method

Place the first six ingredients into the bread machine pan in the order suggested by the bread machine manufacturer. Select the dough cycle and press start.

When the dough is ready, turn it out on a lightly floured surface. Knead lightly until smooth 2 to 3 minutes.

Roll the dough out on a lightly floured surface to form a rectangle approximately 9 inches (23 cm) by 22 inches (55 cm). Mix together the dried fruit, brown sugar and spices. Brush the dough with the melted butter and sprinkle with the fruit mixture. Roll the dough, from the long side, into a Swiss roll shape and cut into 18 equal pieces using a very sharp knife.

Arrange the buns, cut side down, in a lightly buttered 9 inch x 13 inch (23 cm x 33 cm) baking pan. Lightly brush the tops of the buns with melted butter and cover with plastic wrap. Allow the buns to rise in a warm area for about 30-45 minutes. The buns should be touching each other and the dough will be springy.

Note: the ideal place for the buns to rise is in the oven with just the oven light on. Before pre-heating the oven, remove the risen buns and, carefully, remove the plastic wrap. Then, pre-heat the oven to 375°F (190°C, Gas Mark 5).

Bake at 375°F (190°C, Gas Mark 5) for about 20 minutes, until the buns are golden brown and cooked through.

Remove from the oven and cool on a wire rack for about 10 minutes, then drizzle with the sugar glaze.

To make the glaze

In a small saucepan heat the milk and sugar oven medium heat, stirring constantly with a wooden spoon, until the sugar dissolves and it comes to a slight boil. Reduce the heat to low and simmer for 2-3 minutes.

To serve, gently pull the Chelsea buns apart. They can be served warm or cold. They also freeze well.

Servings: 18

Victoria Sponge Cake

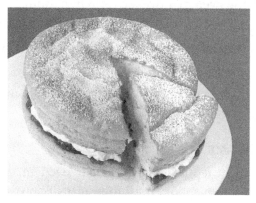

A slice of Victoria Sponge is often served as one of the choices with high tea. You can also offer a Bakewell Tart, Chelsea Bun or Biscuits.

Ingredients

    1 cup (225g) butter, softened
    1½ cups (300g) sugar
    4 eggs
    1 teaspoon (5 mL) almond extract
    2 cups (240g) all purpose flour
    2½ teaspoons (12 mL) baking powder
    ½ teaspoon (2.5 mL) salt
    ½ cup (120 mL) raspberry jam
    2 tablespoons (13g) confectioners sugar
    Whipped Cream Filling
    ½ pint (475 mL) whipping cream
    1 tablespoon (15 mL) sugar
    ¼ teaspoon (1.25 mL) real vanilla

Method

Pre-heat the oven to 350°F (175°C, Gas Mark 4).

Coat two 8 inch (20 cm) round baking pans with non-stick cooking spray and then flour the baking pans as well.

In a large bowl, cream together the butter and the sugar until light and fluffy. Add the eggs one at a time and beat after each addition. Stir in the almond extract.

In a medium bowl or measuring cup, add the flour, baking powder and salt. Mix well.

Fold in flour mixture into the butter mixture until it is just blended. Do not over mix.

Divide the batter equally between the two prepared baking pans.

Bake the sponge cakes at 350°F (175°C, Gas Mark 4) for 20 to 25 minutes or until they are golden brown and a wooden toothpick inserted in the center comes out clean.

Allow the cakes to cool completely on a wire rack.

Carefully remove them from the baking pans. Put the first one on a cake plate and spread the top with the raspberry jam.

Whip The Cream

Pour the cream into a pre-chilled bowl that has steep straight sides. Add the sugar and vanilla. Whip with a hand mixer until the cream forms stiff peaks.

Spread the cream on top of the raspberry jam.

Now put the second sponge layer on top and dust the top with the confectioners sugar.

Servings: 12

CRUMPETS

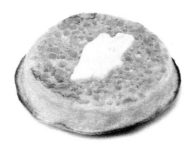

You can't have a book on English baking without a recipe for crumpets but I have to confess this is not something we used to cook ourselves. We just bought them from the local baker. Turns out getting them to look right with the layer of holes on top is kind of tricky.

If you follow the recipe they will taste great but getting them to look right may take a little practice.

INGREDIENTS

3½ cups (820 mL) warm water, divided
1 teaspoon (5 mL) sugar
2 teaspoons (10 mL) active dry yeast
3 cups (360g) all purpose flour
1½ teaspoons (7.5 mL) salt
2 tablespoons (15g) powdered whole milk
1 teaspoon (5 mL) baking soda
2 tablespoons (30 mL) warm water

METHOD

In a measuring cup, combine 1 cup (240 mL) of the warm water and the sugar. Mix until the sugar has dissolved in the warm water. Then, sprinkle the 2 teaspoons (10 mL) of active dry yeast on top of the water and set aside in a warm place for about 10 minutes.

The yeast will foam up. If it doesn't, then the yeast is no longer active and you will need to discard it and start again with some active yeast.

In a large bowl, combine the flour, powdered milk and salt. Mix well.

Make a well in the center of the flour mixture and add the yeast water and the rest of the warm water.

Mix well with a fork to make a thick batter.

Cover the bowl with plastic wrap and set aside in a warm place for about an hour to rise. The mixture won't rise a lot but it will expand and get bubbly.

> *Note: An oven with just the interior light on is a perfect place, and usually warm enough, for the dough to rise.*

Once the batter has risen and is nicely bubbly, combine the baking soda with the 2 tablespoons (30 mL) of water and add it to the dough and mix well.

Cover the bowl again with the plastic wrap and let it stand in a warm place for 15 minutes.

Lightly coat a heavy-bottomed frying pan and the crumpet rings (also called English muffin rings or egg rings) with olive oil. It's easiest to do this with a pastry brush. Pre-heat the frying pan and rings together over medium heat.

> *Note: Getting the temperature just right is a bit of an art. Start with medium heat on your stove and adjust up or down from there based on your results.*

When the frying pan and rings are hot, gently put enough dough in each to come almost to the top of the ring. The dough will rise during cooking.

Cook for 4 to 8 minutes. Bubbles will appear of the entire surface of the crumpet and the dough will start to look dry. At this point, remove the rings and turn the crumpet over. The bottoms should be nicely browned. Cook for an additional 30 seconds to 1 minute to brown the top.

Remove completed crumpets from the pan and cool on a wire rack.

Repeat the process until all the batter is used up.

Crumpets freeze well and can be toasted directly from frozen.

Servings: 24

Crumpets
(Bread Machine Method)

The ingredient quantities are adjusted here to fit most bread machines

Ingredients

    1 cup (240 mL) water
    1 tablespoon (15 mL) olive oil
    ¼ teaspoon (1.25 mL) salt
    1 tablespoon (15 mL) sugar
    1 egg
    2 tablespoons (15g) powdered milk
    1½ cups (180g) all purpose flour
    ½ teaspoon (2.5 mL) baking soda
    2 teaspoons (10 mL) active dry yeast

Method

Place all of the ingredients into the bread machine pan in the order suggested by the bread machine manufacturer. Select the dough cycle and press start.

When the dough cycle is complete, transfer the dough to a large (about 4 cups or 905 mL) measuring cup. Then grease 3 or 4 crumpet rings. Be sure to grease the top and bottom of each ring as well as the inside.

Heat a griddle or heavy skillet over medium heat and grease lightly. Place the crumpet rings on the heated griddle (or skillet) and pour approximately ¼ to ⅓ cup (60 to 80 mL) of the dough (depending on the size of your crumpet rings) into each ring.

Note: this is a very sticky, liquid-type of dough that can be difficult to work with.
Cook the crumpets over medium heat until bubbles form on the top and begin to burst. This takes about 8 to 10 minutes. Carefully remove the crumpet rings and turn the crumpets over to brown the other side. This should take 2-3 minutes.

Repeat the process until you have used up all of the dough.

Crumpets freeze well and can be toasted directly from frozen.

Servings: 12

Custard Tarts

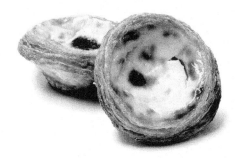

If you're familiar with the British TV series "As Time Goes By" starring Judi Dench and Geoffrey Palmer, you'll remember that the Geoffrey Palmer character loved his custard tarts.

https://en.wikipedia.org/wiki/As_Time_Goes_By_(TV_series)

Ingredients

>   pastry dough, enough for 12 tart shells
>   ¼ cup (60 mL) milk
>   2 eggs
>   1 tablespoon (15 mL) sugar
>   ½ teaspoon (2.5 mL) vanilla
>   1 teaspoon (5 mL) nutmeg, freshly ground

Method

Pre-heat the oven to 400°F (200°C, Gas Mark 6).

On a lightly floured surface, roll out the pastry dough to about ⅛ inch thick and cut out 12 circles. Gently press the pastry circles into muffin tins.

> *Note: If you are pressed for time, you can use pre-made frozen tart shells (thawed).*

Using a whisk, or a fork, beat the eggs, sugar and milk together until well combined. Add the vanilla and stir well.

Pour, or ladle, the egg mixture into tart shells and sprinkle with the freshly grated nutmeg.

Bake the tarts at 400°F (200°C, Gas Mark 6) for 20 minutes or until custard is set and pastry is cooked through. Remove the tarts from the oven and allow to cool completely on a wire rack.

VARIATIONS

Try adding some slices of fresh strawberries, kiwi or peach on top of your tarts.

You can also use this recipe to make one large flan which you decorate with fresh fruit then cut into slices.

Servings: 12

Dundee Cake

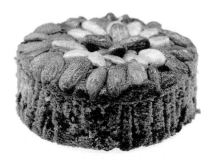

Cake and Scotch whiskey - can it get any better?

Ingredients

    1 cup (225g) butter, softened
    1⅓ cups (240g) packed brown sugar
    4 eggs
    2 cups (240g) all purpose flour
    1 teaspoon (5 mL) baking powder
    1 cup (150g) raisins
    1 cup (150g) currants
    ¾ cup (115g) mixed candied peel
    1 tablespoon (15 mL) grated orange peel
    1 tablespoon (15 mL) grated lemon peel
    ¾ cup (105g) whole blanched almonds
    2 tablespoons (30 mL) corn syrup
    ½ cup (120 mL) Scotch whiskey

Method

Coat an 8 inch (20 cm) spring-form pan with non-stick cooking spray and set aside.

In a medium bowl, cream together the butter with sugar until light and fluffy.

Add eggs one at a time and beat well after each addition.

In a large bowl, mix together the flour, baking powder, raisins, currants, peel and lemon and orange rinds. Ensure that all of the fruit is well-coated with the flour.

Stir the butter mixture into the flour and fruit mixture and mix until well combined. Pour the batter into the prepared spring-form pan, using a spatula to scrape all of the batter out of the bowl.

Arrange the whole almonds in concentric circles over the entire top of the batter. Then press the almonds lightly into the batter.

Place a loaf pan filled with very hot water in the oven and pre-heat the oven to 300°F (150°C, Gas Mark 2).

Bake the cake at 300°F 150°C, Gas Mark 2) for 2 to 2½ hours or until it is a deep golden color and a wooden toothpick inserted in centre comes out clean.

Allow the cake to cool on a wire rack for 5 minutes before removing it from the spring-form pan. Brush the cake with the corn syrup and then allow it to cool completely on the wire rack.

Soak a large piece of cheesecloth (enough to completely enclose the cake) in half of the whiskey and wrap it around the cake. Brush the cake with the remaining whiskey and wrap tightly in aluminum foil.

Refrigerate the cake for at least a week before serving.

> *Note: you can refrigerate it for up to a month before serving if you'd like to make it well in advance.*

Servings: 14

English Bath Buns
(Bread Machine Method)

Like Chelsea Buns, Bath Buns are made with a yeast dough and have a sweet bread taste.

Ingredients

Dough

½ cup (120 mL) water
½ cup (120 mL) milk
2 eggs
1 teaspoon (5 mL) salt
½ cup (115g) butter, softened
2 tablespoons (25g) sugar
4 cups (480g) all purpose flour
1½ tablespoons (22 mL) active dry yeast
Egg Wash
1 egg, lightly beaten with
1 tablespoon (15 mL) water

Almond Topping

¼ cup (50g) sugar
1 cup (140g) chopped almonds

Method

Place all of the dough ingredients into the bread machine in the order suggested by the bread machine manufacturer. Select the dough setting and press start.

When the dough cycle is complete, transfer the dough to a lightly floured surface and knead slightly.

Divide the dough into 24 equal pieces and shape the pieces into smooth balls then flatten them slightly. Place each flattened ball on a greased cookie sheet and cover with plastic wrap.

Let the buns rise in a warm place for about 30 minutes or until doubled in size.

Note: The best place to let dough rise is in an oven with only the oven light turned on.

Once the buns have risen, remove them from the oven and the pre-heat the oven to 375°F (190°C, Gas Mark 5).

While the oven is pre-heating, whisk together the egg and water and brush the tops of the bun with this egg wash.

Note: Don't worry if you have leftover egg wash, you won't need all of it.

Then mix together the chopped almonds and sugar and sprinkle evenly on the buns.

Note: I like to push the chopped almonds slightly into the top of the buns to make sure they'll stick. Just don't push too hard.

Bake the buns at 375°F (190°C, Gas Mark 5) for 20 minutes or until nicely browned and cooked through. Remove them from the cookie sheet and cool on a wire rack.

Servings: 24

English Muffins

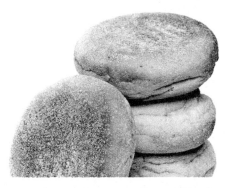

This is a traditional recipe that makes enough muffins for a large family. If you want less you can freeze the leftovers or look at the bread machine recipe that follows this one.

Ingredients

    1 cup (240 mL) milk
    2 tablespoons (25g) sugar
    2 teaspoons (10 mL) active dry yeast
    1 cup (240 mL) warm water
    ¼ cup (55g) butter, melted
    6 cups (720g) all purpose flour
    1 teaspoon (5 mL) salt
    cornmeal, for coating

Method

In a small saucepan, heat the milk over medium-low heat until it comes almost to the boil (small bubble will form). Remove it from the heat and mix in the sugar until it dissolves. Set the saucepan aside and let the milk cool until it is lukewarm.

While the milk is cooling, put the warm water in a small bowl and sprinkle the yeast on top. Let is stand until it is frothy about 10 minutes.

> *Note: If the yeast does not froth then either the water is too hot or too cold or the yeast is no longer active. In that case, throw out the water/yeast mixture and start again.*

In a large bowl combine the milk, yeast mixture, melted butter, 3 cups (360g) of the flour and beat until smooth. Then add the salt and the remaining flour. Knead well until the dough is smooth and elastic.

Transfer the dough to a lightly greased bowl. Turn the dough to ensure it is lightly coated in the grease. Cover the dough with plastic wrap and move it to a warm place to rise until doubled in size - about one hour.

> *Note: The best place to let dough rise is in an oven with only the oven light turned on.*

Once the dough has risen, remove the plastic wrap and turn it out onto a lightly floured surface. Punch down the dough and knead slightly. Roll the dough out to about ½ inch (1.25 cm) thick and cut out rounds with a cookie cutter (about 3 inches or 7.5 cm in diameter). Sprinkle a baking sheet with cornmeal and place the English muffins on the cornmeal. Then dust the tops of muffins with cornmeal as well. Loosely cover the muffins with plastic wrap and allow to rise for about ½ hour.

> *Note: The best place to let the muffins rise is in an oven with only the oven light turned on.*

Heat a heavy skillet (preferably cast iron) over medium-low heat. Spray lightly with non-stick cooking spray.

Gently squeeze each muffin between your palms, being sure to keep them evenly flat, before placing in the hot skillet so they aren't too "puffy". Cook the muffins in the heavy skillet for about 5 to 7 minutes per side. When you turn the muffins, press down on them evenly with a spatula. The muffins will be golden brown on both sides when they are done.

> *Note: Squeezing the muffins before putting them in the pan and then pressing on them after you have turned them will help them maintain the traditional English muffin shape*

You can split the muffins with a fork or serrated knife while they are still warm and serve immediately, or allow to cool on a wire rack.

These English muffins freeze well and can be thawed and toasted later.

Servings: 24

English Muffins
(Bread Machine Method)

If you're bored with bread and want to try something a little different whip up a batch of English muffins in your bread machine.

Ingredients

 1 cup (240 mL) milk, room temperature
 3 tablespoons (40g) butter, room temperature
 1 egg, room temperature
 ½ teaspoon (2.5 mL) salt
 2 teaspoons (10 mL) sugar
 3 cups (360g) all purpose flour
 1½ teaspoons (7.5 mL) dry yeast
 cornmeal, for coating

Method

Place all the ingredients (with the exception of the cornmeal) in the bread machine pan in the order recommended by the manufacturer's instructions.

Select the dough cycle and press start.

When the dough cycle is complete, sprinkle some cornmeal over your work area and remove the dough from the bread machine.

On the prepared surface, pat the dough into a rectangle approximately 1/2 inch (1.25 cm) thick.

Carefully turn the dough so that both sides are lightly coated with the cornmeal.

Using a round cookie cutter (about 3" or 7.5 cm in diameter), cut out 12 to 14 rounds. Rework any trimmings to get the maximum number of muffins.

Place the English muffins on a baking sheet and cover with plastic wrap. Allow them to rise for about 20-30 minutes or until almost doubled in size.

Heat a heavy skillet (preferably cast iron) over medium-low heat. Spray lightly with non-stick cooking spray.

Gently squeeze each muffin between your palms, being sure to keep them evenly flat, before placing in the hot skillet so they aren't too "puffy". Cook the muffins in the heavy skillet for about 5 to 7 minutes per side. When you turn the muffins, press down on them evenly with a spatula. The muffins will be golden brown on both sides when they are down.

Note: squeezing the muffins before putting them in the pan and then pressing on them after you have turned them will help them maintain the traditional English muffin shape.

You can split the muffins with a fork or serrated knife while they are still warm and serve immediately, or allow to cool on a wire rack.

These English muffins freeze well and can be thawed and toasted later.

Servings: 12

Digestive Biscuits

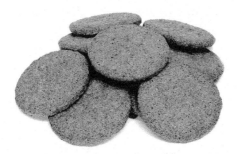

These traditional British biscuits can be served buttered or with cheese. For a sweeter biscuit, brush one side with melted semisweet chocolate after baking.

Ingredients

¾ cup (90g) whole wheat flour
¼ cup (30g) all purpose flour
½ teaspoon (2.5 mL) baking powder
1 tablespoon (15 mL) rolled oats
¼ cup (55g) butter
¼ cup (45g) brown sugar
¼ cup (60 mL) whole milk

Method

Pre-heat the oven to 350°F (175°C, Gas Mark 4) and spray a large baking sheet with non-stick cooking spray.

In a large bowl, combine the whole wheat flour, all-purpose flour and baking powder. Mix well. Add in the oatmeal and mix again.

In a small bowl, cream the butter and brown sugar until well mixed.

Add the creamed butter and sugar to the flour mixture and mix well using a fork to make sure the butter mixture gets well incorporated into the flour mixture.

Add the milk and stir until the mixture forms a thick dough.

Knead the dough on a lightly floured surface until smooth, pliable and no longer sticky.

Carefully roll out dough to about ⅛" thick (.5 cm) and cut into rounds approximately 2½ inches (6.5 cm in diameter with a round cookie cutter.

Note: You may have to re-form any scraps from the first cutting to form the rest of the cookies.

Carefully transfer the biscuits to a greased baking sheet and prick each one well with the tines of a fork.

Note: The biscuits will be fairly fragile so use a very thin spatula to transfer them to the baking sheet.

Bake at 350°F (175°C, Gas Mark 4) for approximately 22 to 25 minutes, or until an even golden brown.

Remove from the oven and allow to cool completely on a wire rack.

Servings: 14

Hot Cross Buns (Bread Machine Method)

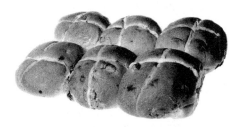

There are lots of hot cross bun recipes around but to me a hot cross bun has a very distinctive taste and that taste is from cardamom, cloves and nutmeg. I know these are a traditional Easter treat but I have never believed you can't have them anytime of the year.

Maybe I have weird taste buds but I like a piece of old cheddar cheese with my hot cross bun - try it.

Ingredients

Dough

1¼ cups (300 mL) milk, room temperature
2 large eggs
1¾ teaspoons (7.5 mL) salt
6 tablespoons (85g) butter, room temperature
¼ cup (45g) light brown sugar, firmly packed
4 cups (480g) all purpose flour
½ teaspoon (2.5 mL) ground cloves
½ teaspoon (2.5 mL) ground nutmeg
2 teaspoon (10 mL) ground cardamom
1 tablespoon (15 mL) baking powder
1 tablespoon (15 mL) active dry yeast
1½ cups (115g) candied mixed peel
Pastry for Crosses
¾ cup (90g) all purpose flour
3 tablespoons (40g) cold butter, cut into small pieces
½ tablespoon (7.5 mL) cold water
Egg Wash
1 large egg
1 tablespoon (15 mL) milk

Glaze

1½ tablespoons (22.5 mL) apricot jam

Method

Add all of the dough ingredients, with the exception of the candied mixed peel, to the bread machine in the order suggested by the manufacturer. Select the dough cycle and press start. Add in the candied mixed peel at the "add-in" beep.

When the dough cycle is complete, transfer the dough to a lightly floured surface and knead slightly. Then divide the dough into 12 equal pieces and shape into balls.

Coat a 9 inch by 13 inch (23 cm by 33 cm) baking dish, preferably glass, with non-stick cooking spray. Place the dough balls in the baking dish, evenly spaced, but not touching. With a very sharp knife, cut a shallow cross into the top of each bun.

Cover the baking dish with plastic wrap and allow buns to rise for about 45 minutes.

Note: The best place to allow dough to rise is in an oven with only the oven light turned on.

Making the Pastry Crosses

While the buns are rising it is time to make the pastry crosses.

Cut the butter into the flour until it is well incorporated. Then, add a little cold water (approximately ½ tablespoon or 7.5 mL) and stir until it makes a thick dough. Add a little more cold water if the dough is too dry.

Roll the dough into a ball and then cut it in half. Cut each half into 6 pieces.

Place the dough in the refrigerator for about 30 minutes. This will make it easier to roll out.

Remove the dough from the refrigerator and roll each piece into a long thin rope. Cut each rope in half and press each piece into the risen buns, forming a cross on the top, being careful not to deflate the buns.

Pre-heat the oven to 350°F (175°C, Gas Mark 4).

Making the Egg Wash

Separate the egg white and yolk. Discard the yolk, or put it aside for another recipe. Whisk together the water and egg white until slightly frothy. Brush the tops of the buns with the egg wash.

Bake the buns at 350°F (175°C, Gas Mark 4) for 20 25 minutes until the are nicely browned.

Remove the buns from the oven and, carefully, transfer them from the baking dish to a wire rack, without separating them. Allow them to cool for about 5 minutes before glazing.

Glazing the Buns

Heat the apricot jam, either on top of the stove or in the microwave, and brush over the still-warm buns to create a nice glaze.

Allow buns to cool completely on a wire rack.

Servings: 12

Madeleines

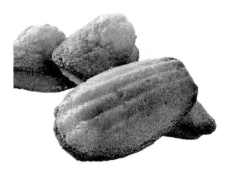

OK, what's a sponge cake from North Eastern France doing in a British baking book?

You'd think the name was a dead giveaway that they aren't British but my mother used to make them quite a bit and I never thought to question their origin. At least not until I started to put this book together and looked them up on Wikipedia. So let's just call this a bonus recipe.

You'll need a special Madeleines pan for this recipe which you can find in kitchen specialty shops.

Ingredients

⅓ cup (75g) butter
3 eggs
1 cup (120g) all purpose flour
½ teaspoon (2.5 mL) baking powder
⅛ teaspoon (1.25 mL) salt
⅔ cup (130g) sugar
1 teaspoon (5 mL) vanilla extract, real, not artificial
powdered sugar, for dusting

Method

Melt the butter and allow it to cool.

With an electric mixer on medium speed, beat the eggs and sugar together until they have approximately tripled in volume. Then add the vanilla extra and beat slightly to incorporate it into the mixture.

In a medium bowl or large measuring cup, mix together the flour, salt and baking powder. Be sure the ingredients are well mixed.

Slowly and carefully fold the flour mixture into the sugar and egg mixture. Be careful not to over mix the batter or it may deflate.

Mix a small amount of the batter into the melted butter. Then slowly fold the butter, about a third of the amount at a time, into the batter. Cover the batter and refrigerate for at least half an hour. The batter should be somewhat firm to the touch.

While the batter is chilling, pre-heat the oven to 375°F (190°C, Gas Mark 5). Generously coat the Madeleine tins with non-stick cooking spray and then dust with flour. Shake off any excess flour. It is essential that the pans are well-greased and floured so that the Madeleines will release easily.

Spoon the chilled batter into the prepared Madeleine pans.

Bake at 375°F (190°C, Gas Mark 5) for 10 to 12 minutes or until the edges are golden brown and the center is slightly springy to the touch. Over-baking will make the Madeleines dry.

Remove the Madeleines from the pans and allow them to cool, smooth side down, on a wire rack. Dust with powdered sugar before serving.

Servings: 24

Maid of Honour Tarts

Ingredients

- 12 unbaked tart shells
- 3 tablespoons (45 mL) Raspberry or cherry jam
- 4 tablespoons (55g) butter
- ¼ cup (50g) sugar
- 1 egg
- ⅓ cup (50g) rice flour
- ¼ teaspoon (1.25 mL) almond flavoring

Method

Pre-heat the oven to 400°F (200°C, Gas Mark 6).

Place one teaspoon of jam in each tart shell and set aside.

In a medium bowl, cream the butter and sugar together until light and fluffy. Add the egg and beat the mixture again. Stir in the rice flour and almond flavoring and mix well.

Place a rounded teaspoonful of the mixture in each tart shell.

Bake the tarts at 400°F (200°C, Gas Mark 6) for about 15 minutes or until pastry and topping are lightly browned.

Remove tarts from the oven and allow them to cool completely on a wire rack.

Servings: 12

Sausage Rolls

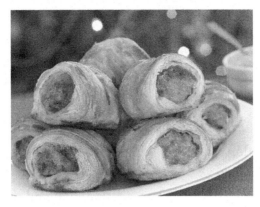

Sausage rolls are great as a snack or serve a couple for lunch with some tomato wedges and some Branston™ pickle.

Ingredients

8 ounces (225g) pork breakfast sausage, cooked
pastry dough, enough for a 1-crust pie

Method

Remove the pork breakfast sausages from their package and cook them over medium heat until they are lightly browned.

Remove the sausages to a plate lined with paper towel to absorb any excess fat and allow the cooked sausages to cool to room temperature and cut each sausage in half.

Pre-heat the oven to 400°F (200°C, Gas Mark 6).

Roll out the pastry dough and cut it into strips just slightly narrower than the length of the sausages (you want a bit of sausage to peak out at each end), and just long enough to wrap around the sausage with a bit of an overlap.

Wrap the pastry around each sausage half and transfer to a slightly greased baking sheet.

Bake at 400°F (200°C, Gas Mark 6) for approximately 10 - 15 minutes or until the pastry is nicely browned.

Remove from oven and cool on a wire rack.

Servings: 24

Pastry Tart Shells

Making really good pastry is an art that deserves a book all to itself. As it so happens my wife Vicky makes the best pastry you have ever tasted. Even my mother admitted Vicky's pastry was better than hers.

Lucky for you Vicky has put everything she knows about making pastry into a book called:

<u>"How To Make Perfect Pastry Every Time"</u>

If you're thinking this is just a plug to get you to buy another book, you're wrong - we would like to give you a copy, free of charge.

Just go to <u>https://fun.geezerguides.com/freebook</u> and once registered you will get an email whenever we have a free promotion for one of our books.

Instant Pot Dundee Cake

Cake and Scotch whiskey - can it get any better?

Ingredients

   1 cup (225g) butter, softened
   1⅓ cups (240g) packed brown sugar
   4 eggs
   2 cups (240g) all purpose flour
   1 teaspoon (5 mL) baking powder
   1 cup (150g) raisins
   1 cup (150g) currants
   ¾ cup (115g) mixed candied peel
   1 tablespoon (15 mL) grated orange peel
   1 tablespoon (15 mL) grated lemon peel
   ¾ cup (105g) whole blanched almonds
   2 tablespoons (30 mL) corn syrup
   ½ cup (120 mL) Scotch whiskey

Method

Coat an 8 inch (20 cm) spring-form pan with non-stick cooking spray and set aside.

In a medium bowl, cream together the butter with sugar until light and fluffy.

Add eggs one at a time and beat well after each addition.

In a large bowl, mix together the flour, baking powder, raisins, currants, peel and lemon and orange rinds. Ensure that all of the fruit is well-coated with the flour.

Stir the butter mixture into the flour and fruit mixture and mix until well combined. Pour the batter into the prepared spring-form pan, using a spatula to scrape all of the batter out of the bowl.

Arrange the whole almonds in concentric circles over the entire top of the batter. Then press the almonds lightly into the batter.

Place 1½ cups (350 mL) of water in the bottom of the Instant Pot insert.

Place the steaming rack in the insert and then place the spring form pan on top of the steaming rack.

Close and lock the lid. Make sure the valve in is the "Sealing" position.

Select the Manual setting and set cooking time for 90 minutes.

When cooking time is complete, allow the pressure to release naturally for 10 minutes and then carefully turn the valve knob to "Venting".

Remove the cake from your Instant Pot and allow it to cool on a wire rack for 5 minutes before removing it from the spring-form pan.

Brush the cake with the corn syrup and then allow it to cool completely on the wire rack.

Soak a large piece of cheesecloth (enough to completely enclose the cake) in half of the whiskey and wrap it around the cake. Brush the cake (still wrapped in the cheesecloth) with the remaining whiskey and wrap tightly in aluminum foil.

Refrigerate the cake for at least a week before serving.

> *Note: you can refrigerate it for up to a month before serving if you'd like to make it well in advance.*

Servings: 14

Air Fryer Sausage Rolls

The Air Fryer recipe for Sausage Rolls is pretty much the same as the regular recipe except you do fewer pieces at a time and it cooks faster.

Also, if you've got just a few leftover sausages and a little bit of leftover pastry, then you've got a quick meal.

Here's how to make these tasty little treat in your Air Fryer. The quantity you make will be up to you, but 4 - 6 sausage rolls will fit nicely in an Air Fryer basket.

Ingredients

Cooked, lightly browned breakfast sausages, cut in half
Pastry (amount will depend on how many sausages you plan to use)

Method

Pre-heat the Air Fryer to 400°F (200°C).

Roll out the pastry dough and cut it into strips just slightly narrower than the length of the sausages (you want a bit of sausage to peak out at each end), and just long enough to wrap around the sausage with a bit of an overlap.

Wrap the pastry strips around each sausage half and gently transfer to the Air Fryer Basket.

Bake at 400°F (200°C) for approximately 5 minutes, check to see if they're browning, and cook for an additional 5 minutes, if necessary.

Spotted Dick

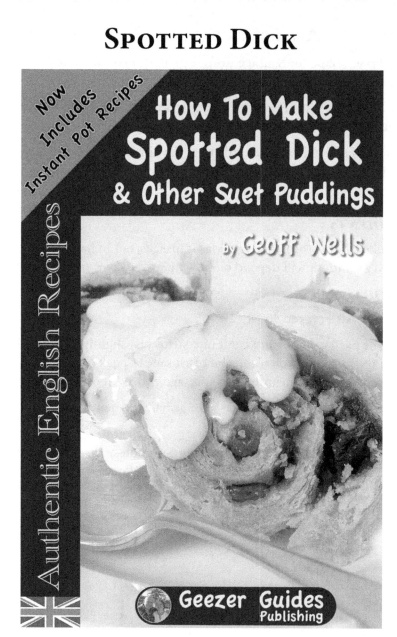

Introduction

Spotted Dick is not the king of suet puddings but it certainly has the most memorable name - at least as far as North Americans are concerned.

Spotted Dicks are often the featured dessert items on British menus and it's not unusual to see many English men and women enjoying their Dicks covered in Bird's custard or Tate & Lyle's Golden Syrup.

FAQ's

What Is Suet?

The secret to making a great Spotted Dick is suet which is just a kind of fat.

Suet is the beef fat that surrounds the kidneys. It has a high melting point between 113°F and 122°F (45°C and 50°C). This is much higher than lard, (pork fat), which has a melting point between 86°F and 104°F (30°C and 40°C). Leaf fat lard, which is the highest grade, has a melting point between 109°F and 118°F (43°C and 48°C). Unfortunately leaf fat lard is rarely available commercially.

But I'm A Vegetarian

Not to worry, although true suet is made from animal fat you can buy a light version made entirely from vegetable fat. This is a commercial product made by Atora that can be used in any suet recipe.

Where Can I Buy Suet?

In Europe suet is readily available at any grocery store. I'm not sure about Australia but I imagine it is much like Canada where you can buy it if you ask the butcher to get it for you. In the US, where all the food is controlled by just a few giant corporations, you may have difficulty finding it in any store. Fortunately it is readily available online and you can find links at our web site https://ebooks.geezerguides.com/products-from-our-books/

From The Butcher

If you are lucky enough to find a butcher that sells fresh suet you might be able to persuade him to prepare it for you - otherwise you can do it yourself.

Trim the pink connective tissue leaving just the pure white fat. Now chop the fat as finely as you can. Your butcher would run it through the meat grinder and if you have a home unit that would be perfect. A blender is not a good choice as you want the suet chopped not turned into a paste.

Substitutes for Suet

Real suet can be difficult to find in North America. If you are not able to obtain real suet you can substitute:

- ❖ the same amount of lard, frozen and shredded or
- ❖ the same amount of vegetable shortening, frozen and shredded or
- ❖ a package of Atora™ from Amazon
- ❖ http://amzn.to/2vXHD4d

What Is A Steamed Pudding?

As the name suggests a steamed pudding is cooked by steam rather than putting it in a dry oven. Usually, but not always, the pudding basin is lined with the suet crust, filled with meat or fruit, and closed with a suet crust top. The top is then covered with greasproof paper (wax or parchment paper is the closest US equivalent) and a cloth. Then the basin is lowered into a saucepan full of boiling water and cooked for about 3 hours.

What's A Pudding Cloth?

This is something cooks would fashion from an old bed sheet or similar material. It is laid on top of the pudding and tied under the lip of the basin with string. The four corners of the cloth are then raised on top and tied together. This provides a handle to remove the basin from the boiling water.

What Is A Pudding Basin?

If you go to our website you can see pictures of pudding basins which should make the idea clear. Basically it is a ceramic bowl with a lip around the edge. When you cover the top of your pudding with greasproof paper and a cloth you hold them on with a piece of string tied under the lip.

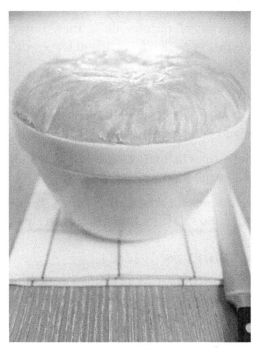

Typical Pudding Basin

Must I Use A Pudding Basin?

No, a Spotted Dick is steamed without a basin but any meat or fruit pudding is cooked in a container. Any ceramic bowl or basin with a lip around the edge will work.

You can also make individual suet puddings in ramekins.

How Much Cooking Water Do I Use?

Lower the basin into the saucepan containing about half a pot of water. The water level should be almost to the top of the basin but not covering it.

Bring the water to a boil and maintain the water level throughout the cooking process. Check every half hour or so and replenish any lost water by adding boiling water.

The saucepan should have a well fitting lid.

Self-Raising Flour

I think it is safe to say that most suet recipes you will find come from England, (most, not all). It's also a fair bet that many of those recipes will call for self-raising flour because that is more the norm than in North America. Even though self-raising flour is available in the US and Canada, North American recipes will typically specify all purpose flour. There is nothing magical about self-raising flour. It is just flour that has salt and leavening agents added.

To make your own self-raising flour just add 1½ teaspoons of baking powder and ¼ teaspoon of salt to 1 cup of all purpose flour. Make sure you mix it well.

Alternatively you can add one teaspoon of cream of tartar, ½ teaspoon of bicarbonate of soda and ¼ teaspoon of salt which will work just as well.

That being said all the recipes in this book are designed for the North American market and so use all purpose flour.

Obviously if you are in England and normally use self-raising flour just leave out the baking powder and salt from the suet crust recipes.

Measuring Ingredients

Most of the books in this series are more about the method and ingredients of the recipes rather than exact quantities. This book is a little different as it is all about baking and baking just won't work unless you get the chemistry right.

These are my mother's recipes, modified for the North American measuring system. I have also changed any reference to self-raising flour because it is not widely available here.

Basic Suet Crust

A suet crust is just a type of pastry but instead of baking it in an oven you boil or steam it. The result is more like a dumpling than a pie crust. In fact what I consider "real" dumplings are always made with suet. If you normally use Bisquik® for your dumplings give my suet dumpling recipe a try.

Suet pudding is a delicious English tradition found in both meat and fruit dishes. It can be eaten as is or covered with various toppings depending on if you are preparing an entrée or a dessert.

The basic recipe for a suet crust is 1 part suet to 1½ parts flour Since this is self-raising flour you will need to add 1½ teaspoons of baking powder and ¼ teaspoon of salt to every cup of all purpose flour.

A Few Tips

There are a few tips I want to share that will help make your suet puddings as good as they can be.

Start with your suet at room temperature. In other words take it out of the fridge an hour or so before you begin using it.

Suet pastry expands quite a bit as it cooks so be sure to allow for this. Fill pudding basins only two-thirds full to allow room for expansion.

Before cooking baked suet dishes, always make sure the oven is preheated to the correct temperature.

When steaming puddings make sure the water is boiling before the pudding is placed in the steamer or pan. Always top up the level with boiling water from a kettle.

How To Steam

Select a saucepan that is a little bit larger than your pudding basin. Half fill the saucepan with water and gentle lower your basin into the water. The water level should be just below the rim of the basin. Adjust the water level so that the boiling water will not spill on top of your pudding.

Use a tight fitting lid and adjust the water level every half hour.

Using A Steamer

A steamer works great for Spotted Dicks and Roly-polys. It's also a good choice if you make individual puddings in ramekins.

Using an Instant Pot

We now use an Instant Pot whenever we make a steamed pudding. It's just easier and more convenient.

It's much faster and we don't have to worry about the water level.

If you don' yet have an Instant Pot don't let that stop you from making these puddings but when you do get one be sure to try the Instant Pot methods that I have added.

Savoury Suet Pastry

Use this recipe for all your savoury meat and cheese puddings. Use ¾ of the dough to line the bottom and sides of your basin and the remaining ¼ for the pastry lid.

Ingredients

    1½ cups (180g) flour
    1 tablespoon (15 mL) baking powder
    ¾ teaspoon (4 mL) salt
    ¼ teaspoon (1.25 mL) pepper
    1 cup (125g) suet (see Page 186 for alternatives)
    8 - 10 tablespoons (40-50 mL) cold water

Method

In a medium bowl, mix together the flour, baking powder, salt and pepper. Mix well with a fork to make sure the ingredients are well combined.

Cut in the suet, using a pastry blender, until the mixture looks like a coarse meal.

Trickle the cold water over the dry ingredients and mix with a fork until it begins to form a dough. Then, knead the dough until it is well formed and still a little sticky.

Sweet Suet Pastry

Use this recipe for all your sweet and fruit puddings. For filled fruit pudding use ¾ of the dough to line the bottom and sides of your basin and the remaining ¼ for the pastry lid.

If you're making a rolled pudding like a Spotted Dick or Roly-poly, roll the pastry to a rectangle approximately 8 inches by 12 inches. Add your filling and roll up to form an 8 inch finished length.

Ingredients

    1½ cups (180 g) all purpose flour
    ⅓ cup (65g) sugar
    1 tablespoon (15 mL) baking powder
    ¾ teaspoon (4 mL) salt
    1 cup (125g) <u>suet</u>, finely chopped (see Page 186 for alternatives)
    8 - 10 tablespoons (40-50 mL) milk

Method

In a medium bowl, mix together the flour, sugar, baking powder and salt. Mix well with a fork to make sure the ingredients are well combined.

Cut in the suet, using a pastry blender, until the mixture looks like a coarse meal.

Trickle the milk over the dry ingredients and mix with a fork until it begins to form a dough. Then, knead the dough until it is well formed and still a little sticky.

Spotted Dick

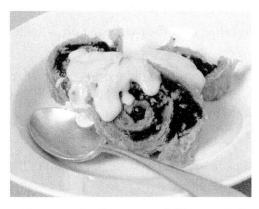

This recipe comes with a couple of suggested fillings. As long as you keep the measurements about the same, feel free to experiment with different types of fillings.

Ingredients

1 recipe sweet suet pastry (see Page 192)

Filling #1

¾ cup (115g) currants
1 small cooking apple, peeled, cored and diced
⅓ cup (60g) brown sugar
½ large lemon, zest only

Filling #2

¼ cup (40g) currants
¼ cup (40g) craisins (dried cranberries)
¼ cup (30g) walnuts
¼ cup (40g) dried mixed fruit
⅓ cup (60g) brown sugar, packed

Your Filling

It's okay to experiment. As long as you keep the quantities about the same you can mix up the filling ingredients. For example, I used raisins instead of currants, chopped almonds instead of walnuts, some chopped candied peel instead of the dried mix fruit … you get the idea.

Method

In a medium bowl, mix all the filling ingredients together making sure that the brown sugar is well distributed throughout the fruit and nuts. Set aside.

On a lightly floured surface, roll out the sweet suet pastry to form a rectangle approximately 8 inches by 12 inches (20 cm x 30 cm).

Evenly distribute the filling over the pastry and press the filling lightly into the pastry.

Roll up the pastry, as tightly as possible, from the smaller end. For example, start from the edge that is 8 inches (20 cm) wide so when you are finished you have a Spotted Dick that is 8 inches (20 cm) long.

Seal the ends and the seam by pinching them together.

Wrap the Spotted Dick in several layers of aluminum foil, twisting the ends to seal the package.

Steam the pudding for 2 hours.

Remove the completed Spotted Dick from the steamer and carefully unwrap. It will be very hot.

Slice off individual portions and serve with Tate & Lyle's Golden Syrup or Bird's dessert custard.

Servings: 6

Suet Dumplings

Add dumplings to soups and stews during the last 10 - 20 minutes of cooking.

You can get creative and fill the centres with meat or cheese. Even boiling them in water and using them as a course on their own.

Try filling them with apples and raisins then cover with custard as a dessert.

Ingredients

- ½ cup (120g) flour
- ¼ cup (30g) shredded suet (see Page 186 for alternatives)
- ¾ teaspoon (3.75 mL) baking powder
- ⅛ teaspoon (1.25 mL) salt
- 5 tablespoons (75 mL) cold water, approximately

Method

Put the flour, suet, baking powder and salt in a small bowl and mix well. Add just enough cold water to make the dough pliable but not sticky.

If it's too sticky add a little more flour.

Put a little flour on your hands and divide the dough into 8 pieces then roll them into balls.

About 10 - 20 minutes before your stew is done, drop the balls into the simmering liquid. Keep covered and cook gently until done. Turn them over half way through the process.

Servings: 4

Suggestions

You can add some interest by experimenting with various herbs added to your dough. Check out the Atora website for more dumpling recipes.

Apple and Blackberry Suet Pudding

This was my favorite fruit pudding combination but unfortunately I've never been able to find wild blackberries in North America with the intense flavour as those we used to pick on the common behind our house in England.

Ingredients

1 recipe <u>sweet suet pastry</u> (see Page 192)

Filling

2 large cooking apples, cored, peel and sliced

1½ cups (190g) blackberries

⅓ cup (65g) sugar

Method

Roll out the sweet suet pastry and line a 1½ pint (700 mL) pudding basin with three-quarters of the pastry, reserving one-quarter for the lid.

In a medium bowl, toss together the apple slices, blackberries and sugar. Ladle the fruit and sugar mixture into the pastry-lined pudding basin.

Wet the edges of the pastry lid and then pinch the edges to seal the lid.

Cover the top of the pudding basin with waxed paper and a pudding cloth, tie securely with string and gather any excess pudding cloth over the top of the basin.

Steam for 2½ to 3 hours.

Serve with Bird's custard, heavy cream or ice cream.

Servings: 6

Suggestions

You can use many fruit combinations to make delicious puddings. Some of my favorite filings are plum, red and black currents, rhubarb, peach and gooseberry.

Carrot-Raisin Suet Pudding

This pudding is molded by the basin and turned out on a plate to serve. Cut generous slices and serve them with Bird's custard.

Ingredients

- 2 medium carrots, coarsely grated
- 2 medium apples, peeled, cored and finely chopped
- 1 medium potato, peeled and finely chopped
- 1 cup (125g) suet, chopped (see Page 186 for alternatives)
- 1 cup (200g) sugar
- ⅓ cup (80 mL) orange juice
- 1 egg, beaten
- 1 teaspoon (5 mL) vanilla
- 1½ cups (180g) all purpose flour
- 1½ teaspoons (7.5 mL) baking soda
- 1 teaspoon (5 mL) cinnamon
- 1 teaspoon (5 mL) nutmeg, freshly grated
- ½ teaspoon (2.5 mL) ground cloves
- ½ teaspoon (2.5 mL) salt
- 1 cup (175g) dates, chopped
- 1 cup (150g) raisins

Method

Grease a 2 pint (950 mL) pudding basin.

In a large bowl, combine the carrots, apples, potato and suet. Mix well.

In a large measuring cup, combine the sugar, orange juice, egg, and vanilla. Mix well and stir into the carrot mixture.

In a medium bowl, combine the flour, baking soda, cinnamon, nutmeg, cloves, and salt. Mix well and stir into the carrot mixture.

Fold the dates and raisins into the carrot mixture.

Pour the batter into the greased pudding basin.

Cover the top of the basin with waxed paper and then a pudding cloth. Secure the pudding cloth with string and gather any excess cloth over the top.

Steam the pudding for 3½ hours.

Servings: 8

Christmas Plum Pudding

Traditionally our Christmas puddings contained several six-penny pieces but, although we all survived, this is not a tradition I would recommend.

Ingredients

- 1¼ cups (150g) all purpose flour
- ½ teaspoon (2.5 mL) baking soda
- 1 teaspoon (5 mL) salt
- 1¼ cups (190g) Sultana raisins
- 1¼ cups (190g) seedless raisins
- 1 cup (150g) currants
- 1 cup (75g) mixed peel, chopped
- 1 cup (95g) maraschino cherries
- 1 cup (110g) blanched almonds, chopped
- 2 tablespoons (15g) all purpose flour
- ½ cup (115g) butter
- 1¼ cups (225g) brown sugar, firmly packed
- 4 eggs, beaten
- 2 tablespoons (30 mL) molasses
- 1½ cups (135g) dry bread crumbs
- ½ cup (120 mL) brandy
- 1 teaspoon (5 mL) cinnamon
- ½ teaspoon (2.5 mL) nutmeg
- ½ teaspoon (2.5 mL) ground cloves
- 1½ cups (185g) suet, finely chopped (see Page 186 for alternatives)
- ⅔ cup (160 mL) milk

Method

In a medium bowl or measuring cup, combine the flour, baking soda and salt. Set aside.

In a medium bowl, mix together the raisins, currants, peel, cherries, nuts and 2 tablespoons (15g) of flour. Toss well so that the flour coats all the other ingredients. Set aside.

In a large bowl cream together the butter and brown sugar until light and fluffy.

Beat the eggs well and add to the butter and sugar mixture. Then add the molasses, bread crumbs, brandy, spices and suet. Mix well.

Add in the floured fruit and nut mixture and mix well.

Add the flour, baking soda and salt mixture alternately with the milk and mix well.

Grease the pudding molds well and fill about 2/3rds full as the puddings will rise.

Cover with waxed paper and a pudding cloth tied with string.

Steam for 4 to 5 hours.

Serve warm.

Note: the pudding can be reheated by steaming for about 1½ to 2 hours.

Serve with a brandy or rum sauce which you can light just before bringing to the table. The flame maybe difficult to see unless you turn out the lights.

Servings: 8

> *Note: Christmas puddings are traditionally made months ahead and develop their flavour the longer you keep them.*

FIGGY PUDDING

This is a very simple recipe for figgy pudding. It's fun to sometimes switch things around and serve a light entrée with the dessert as the feature.

INGREDIENTS

¾ cup (95g) suet (see Page 186 for alternatives)
¾ cup (135g) brown sugar, packed
3 eggs
¼ cup (60 mL) cream sherry
1 cup (150g) figs, chopped
¼ cup (60 mL) molasses
1 teaspoon (5 mL) ground cinnamon
1½ cups (135g) dried bread crumbs
1 teaspoon (5 mL) vanilla

METHOD

Generously grease a 2 pint (950 mL) pudding basin and then coat with white sugar.

In a large bowl, combine the suet and brown sugar and mix well.

Add the eggs, vanilla and molasses and beat until well mixed.

Add the dried bread crumbs and cinnamon and mix until combined.

Add the cream sherry and mix just enough to make sure the sherry is well incorporated into the mixture.

Fold in the chopped figs.

> *Note: If you are using dried figs, rehydrate them by putting them in a small saucepan covered with water. Bring them to a boil, reduce heat and allow them to simmer for about 15 minutes. Pour off the excess liquid, allow the figs to cool and then coarsely chop them.*

Pour the completed batter into the prepared pudding basin. Cover the basin with some waxed paper and then a cloth. Tie with string and then lift the excess cloth over the top of the bowl and pin (this will be helpful when lifting the pudding in and out of the steaming pan).

Place the pudding in a pan large enough to hold the bowl with room left over. Fill the pan with hot water about three-quarters up the pudding basin. Cover the pan and bring the water to a boil over medium-high heat. Once the water is boiling, reduce heat to low and let the pudding steam for 3 hours.

Note: be sure to check the water every hour or so and add additional, boiling water as required.

When pudding is done, remove from basin and invert on a serving plate.

Serve warm with dessert custard.

Servings: 8

Ginger Pudding

If you want to be really decadent you can warm some ginger marmalade and use that as a topping instead of the syrup.

Ingredients

    1 cup (120g) all purpose flour
    1½ teaspoons (7.5 mL) ground ginger
    ¼ teaspoon (1.25 mL) baking soda
    ½ cup (120 mL) milk
    2 tablespoons (30 mL) Tate & Lyle's Golden Syrup
    2 tablespoons (30 mL) preserved ginger, chopped
    1 egg
    1½ cups (135g) bread crumbs
    1 tablespoon (15 mL) brown sugar
    1½ cups (190g) <u>suet</u> (see Page 186 for alternatives)

Method

In a small bowl, combine the flour, ground ginger and baking soda. Mix well and set aside.

In a small saucepan, heat the milk just to the simmering point, remove from heat and add the golden syrup and the beaten egg. Mix well.

> *Note: golden corn syrup may be substituted if you cannot get Tate & Lyle's Golden Syrup*

Stir in the bread crumbs, sugar, suet and chopped, preserved ginger. Add the flour mixture and stir to combine everything well.

Pour the completed mixture into a well greased 2 pint (950 mL) pudding basin.

Cover the top of the basin with waxed paper and then a pudding cloth. Secure the pudding cloth with string and gather any excess cloth over the top.

Steam the pudding for 2 hours.

Servings: 4

Jam Roly-Poly

This is a simple recipe that makes a wonderful dessert. It's very easy to make variations by changing the kind of jam or marmalade you use.

Ingredients

>1 recipe <u>sweet suet pastry</u> (see Page 192)
>5 - 6 tablespoons (75 - 90 mL) jam of your choice

Method

On a lightly floured surface, roll out the suet pastry to create a rectangle approximately 8 inches (20 cm) by 10 inches (25 cm).

Spread the rolled dough with the jam of your choice. The traditional choices are often raspberry or strawberry jam.

Spread the jam to about ½ an inch (1.25 cm) away from the edges.

Use some cold water to slightly wet the edges of the pastry. Then, roll up the pastry, from the shorter edge and seal the edges and seam.

Wrap the roly-poly well in 2 or 3 layers of aluminum foil and steam for 1½ hours.

Serve this dessert hot. Cut it into slices and serve with a dessert custard. It's also nice served with ice cream.

Baked Roly-Poly

This recipe can also be baked. In order to bake it, pre-heat your oven to 400°F (200°C, Gas Mark 6).

Coat a baking dish with non-stick cooking spray.

Bake at 400°F (200°C, Gas Mark 6) for 30-35 minutes, or until golden brown.

>*Note: DO NOT wrap it in foil as you would for steaming.*

Servings: 6

Leicestershire Pudding

This pudding is a good candidate to try as individual servings made in ramekins. Cook in a vegetable steamer for 1½ - 2 hours.

Ingredients

    1½ cups (225g) raisins, seedless
    1 cup (120g) all purpose flour
    ¾ cup (95g) <u>suet</u>, chopped (see Page 186 for alternatives)
    2 eggs, beaten
    1 teaspoon (5 mL) grated lemon peel
    1 teaspoon (5 mL) nutmeg, freshly grated
    2 tablespoons (30 mL) brandy
    milk as needed

Method

Grease a 1½ pint (700 mL) pudding basin.

In a large bowl, combine the raisins, flour and suet and mix well. Mix together the raisins, flour and suet in a bowl.

Add the beaten eggs, lemon peel, nutmeg and brandy. Mix well.

Knead in enough milk to produce a firm dough and transfer the mixture into the greased pudding basin.

Cover with waxed paper and a pudding cloth tied with string.

Steam the pudding for 4 hours.

Serve with whipped cream or custard.

Servings: 6

Lemony Sussex Pond Pudding

This pudding is from the county of Sussex and contains a whole lemon. During the long cooking time the lemon flavour infuses the butter and brown sugar which makes a thick lemon caramel.

Be sure to scrape out the centre of the lemon when you serve it. You can, of course, eat the candied skin if you wish.

Grocery store lemons are covered in wax so buy your lemons for this dish from an organic supplier.

Ingredients

    1 recipe sweet suet pastry (see Page 192)
    zest of 1 lemon
    ½ cup (45g) breadcrumbs

Filling

    ¾ cup (170g) cold butter, cut into small cubes
    ¾ cup (135g) brown sugar
    1 large whole lemon, (this is a 2nd lemon with the skin intact)

Method

Start by adding the zest of one lemon and the breadcrumbs to the sweet suet pastry recipe.

Grease a 1½ quart (1.5 L) pudding basin.

Roll out the sweet suet pastry and line the pudding basin with the pastry. Reserve enough pastry to make a lid for after you have filled the pudding.

Put the lemon on a hard surface and roll your hand over it. This will help to release the juice. Prick the lemon all over with a fork or toothpick then add half the sugar, butter and whole lemon to the centre of the pudding. Place the remaining sugar and butter around the edge of the lemon.

Wet the edges of the suet pastry lid and place on top. Pinch the edges to seal.

Cover the top of the basin with waxed paper and then a pudding cloth. Secure the pudding cloth with string and gather any excess cloth over the top.

Steam the pudding for 3 hours.

Serve with custard, heavy cream or ice cream.

Servings: 6

Middlesex Pond Pudding

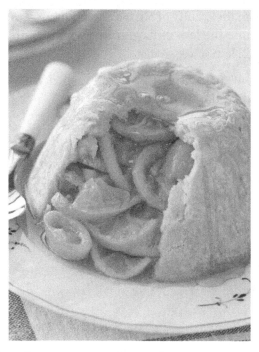

You will notice that this is very similar to the previous recipe for the Sussex Pond Pudding. Middlesex is the county I was born in so, as this was my variation, I named it thus but this is the only place you will find anything called a Middlesex Pond Pudding.

Ingredients

    1 recipe sweet suet pastry (see Page 192)
    zest of ½ orange
    ½ cup (45g) breadcrumbs

Filling

    1 small lemon, thinly sliced
    1 small lime, thinly sliced
    1 small orange, thinly sliced
    2 tablespoons (15g) all purpose flour
    ¾ cup (135g) brown sugar
    ½ cup (150g) cold butter, cut into small cubes

Method

Start by adding the zest of one lemon and the breadcrumbs to the sweet suet pastry recipe.

Grease a 1½ quart (1.5 L) pudding basin.

Roll out the sweet suet pastry and line the pudding basin with the pastry. Reserve enough pastry to make a lid for after you have filled the pudding.

In a medium bowl toss the lemon, lime and orange slices with the 2 tablespoons (15g) of all purpose flour.

To make the filling, create layers starting with 2 tablespoons (25g) of the brown sugar, 3 or 4 cubes of butter and a few slices of lemon, lime and orange. Continue with these layers until you've used up all of the filling ingredients.

Wet the edges of the suet pastry lid and place on top. Pinch the edges to seal.

Cover the top of the basin with waxed paper and then a pudding cloth. Secure the pudding cloth with string and gather any excess cloth over the top.

Steam the pudding for 3 hours.

Servings: 6

TREACLE PUDDING

If you have a sweet tooth you'll be sure to like this. Like the Leicestershire Pudding this works well as individual servings made in ramekins. Cook in a vegetable steamer for about an hour.

INGREDIENTS

¼ cup (60 mL) dark treacle, substitute molasses if you can't find treacle
¼ cup (60 mL) Tate & Lyle's golden syrup, substitute corn syrup if you can't find Tate & Lyle's
¼ teaspoon (1.25 mL) cinnamon
2 cups (240g) all purpose flour
3 teaspoons (15 mL) baking powder
1 cup (125g) suet, finely chopped (see Page 186 for alternatives)
⅓ cup (60g) brown sugar
⅓ cup (65g) white sugar
⅔ cup (160 mL) milk
2 eggs, beaten

METHOD

Grease a 1½ pint (700 mL) pudding basin.

Note: make sure to grease the basin well or the treacle might stick.

Pour the treacle and golden syrup into the base of the pudding basin.

In a medium bowl combine the flour, cinnamon and baking powder and mix well. Cut in the suet with a pastry blender until the mixture resembles a coarse meal.

Add both the white and brown sugar to the flour mixture and stir well.

In a medium bowl, combine the milk and beaten eggs.

Slowly pour the egg mixture into the flour mixture and stir until all ingredients are well combined and make a soft, sticky dough.

Carefully spoon the dough into the pudding basin being careful not to disturb the treacle too much.

Cover the top of the basin with waxed paper and then a pudding cloth. Secure the pudding cloth with string and gather any excess cloth over the top.

Steam the pudding for 2 hours.

Allow the pudding to cool on a wire rack for 5 minutes and then turn the pudding out on a plate, allowing the treacle to dribble down the sides.

Servings: 6

Bonus Recipe - Mincemeat

I have included a mincemeat recipe because mincemeat is made with suet. Commercial mincemeat is surprisingly expensive and not nearly as good as homemade. This recipe is for a small quantity that you would use for a pie. If you wish you can make a big batch and store it for a year or more.

You should make it at least two weeks before you plan to use it so that the flavours have a chance to mature.

Ingredients

1 cup (125g) finely chopped beef <u>suet</u> (see Page 186 for alternatives)
2 granny smith apples, unpeeled, cored and finely chopped
1 cup (150g) raisins
¾ cup (115g) currants
½ cup (75g) sultanas
½ cup (90g) packed dark brown sugar
¼ cup (20g) candied peel (lemon/orange)
zest and juice of ½ a fresh lemon
zest and juice of one orange
1½ teaspoons (7.5 mL) freshly grated nutmeg
½ teaspoon (2.5 mL) ground cloves
¼ teaspoon (1.25 mL) mace
½ teaspoon (2.5 mL) cinnamon
¼ cup (60 mL) brandy or dark rum

Method

In a bowl, combine everything except the brandy or rum. Mix well.

Transfer the mixture to a saucepan and heat until the suet has completely melted and the mixture is heated through.

Remove from heat, cool, then stir in the brandy. Pack into a 2 - 2 cup (475 mL) jars and refrigerate.

Of course if you properly sterilize and seal your jars the mincemeat will keep for years without refrigeration. After all mincemeat was originally a way to preserve meat.

Cheese and Leek Suet Pudding

I've always thought that leeks are a much under used vegetable. Try these next two recipes for something a little different.

Ingredients

1 recipe savoury suet pastry (see Page 191)

Filling

3 tablespoons (40g) butter
1 pound (450g) leeks
2 tablespoons (15g) all purpose flour
1 cup (100g) sharp cheddar cheese, shredded
¼ cup (60 mL) water
1 teaspoon (5 mL) dried thyme
sea salt, to taste
freshly ground black pepper, to taste

Method

Cut the leeks in half, lengthwise and clean well. Remove the tougher green pieces and slice.

In a large skillet, melt the butter over low heat and add the leeks. Cook for about 10 minutes or until soft. Sprinkle the flour over the leeks, mix well and continue to cook, over low heat, for another 2 minutes.

Slowly add the milk, stirring constantly. Then add the grated cheese and stir well to combine.

When the mixture begins to thicken, remove from heat and stir in the salt and pepper to taste. Set aside and allow the mixture to cool completely.

Once the cheese and leek filling has cooled, grease a 2 pint (950 mL) pudding basin, roll out the suet pastry and line the pudding basin with the pastry. Ladle the filling into the basin and then cover with a pastry lid.

Cover the top of the basin with waxed paper and then a pudding cloth. Secure the pudding cloth with string and gather any excess cloth over the top.

Steam the pudding for 2 hours.

Servings: 4

Ham and Leek Suet Pudding

After you have tried these two leek recipes, why not combine them for a third variation.

Ingredients

1 recipe savoury suet pastry (see Page 191)

Filling

12 ounces (340g) cooked ham
1 leek
1½ tablespoons (25g) butter
1½ tablespoons (11g) all purpose flour
1 cup (240 mL) chicken stock
2 sprigs fresh thyme
pepper, to taste

Method

Cut the cooked ham into small cubes. Wash the leek well and remove the tough green top of the leek. Then cut the leek into thin slices.

In a medium saucepan, melt the butter over medium heat and cook the leek slices until tender. Sprinkle the flour over the leeks and stir well.

Slowly add the hot chicken stock, stirring constantly. Continue stirring, over medium heat, until the mixture comes to a boil and begins to thicken.

Reduce heat and add the thyme, cream and ham.

Stir well and simmer for about 5 minutes.

Remove from heat and set aside to cool.

Once the ham and leek filling has cooled, grease a 2 pint (950 mL) pudding basin, roll out the suet pastry and line the pudding basin with the pastry. Ladle the filling into the basin and then cover with a pastry lid.

Cover the top of the basin with waxed paper and then a pudding cloth. Secure the pudding cloth with string and gather any excess cloth over the top.

Steam the pudding for 2 hours.

Servings: 4

Steak and Kidney Pudding

Of all the meals I enjoyed growing up this was my favorite. I truly believe there isn't a better tasting meal to be had. Please try it at least once, exactly as I present it.

I know how Americans gag at the thought of eating kidney but before you do check out what goes into a hot dog.

http://www.dailymail.co.uk/news/article-2175655/So-really-ingredients-really-sausage-Read-eat-frankfurter-again.html

If you really can't bring yourself to try it leave it in large pieces and remove it before serving. This way you at least get the benefit of the flavour in your gravy. Trust me - this will be the best gravy you have ever tasted.

Ingredients

1 recipe savoury suet pastry (see Page 191)

Filling

3 - 4 lb (1.3 - 1.8 Kg) blade or top sirloin roast
⅓ beef kidney
1 large onion
4 medium carrots
½ teaspoon (2.5 mL) salt
2 tablespoons (30 mL) of Bovril™
2 tablespoons (15g) corn starch

Method

Cut the roast into 1 inch (2.5 cm) cubes and be sure to remove any fat, skin or gristle. Cut the kidney into bite size pieces or ½ dozen pieces if you don't plan to eat it.

Put the cubes in a large saucepan with a heavy bottom. Over a fairly high heat toss the cubes around in the saucepan until all the meat is seared and no red is visible.

Add cold water until the water is almost at the level of the meat. DO NOT add too much water, it will dilute the taste.

Chop the onion and add it to the pot. Peel the carrots and chop them into 1 inch (2.5 cm) pieces. Add them to the pot. Add the Bovril™.

Bring the beef mixture to a simmer and cook for 30 minutes or until the carrots are just starting to soften. Remove from heat and drain the gravy into another saucepan. Don't overcook it.

Mix the cornstarch with just enough water to make a thin paste. Use as little water as possible to make the cornstarch workable.

Bring the gravy to a simmer and slowly add the cornstarch until the gravy is the consistency of cooking oil.

Once the beef and kidney filling has cooled, grease a 2 pint (950 mL) pudding basin, roll out the suet pastry and line the pudding basin with the pastry. Ladle the filling into the basin and add ¼ cup (60 mL) of the gravy.

Don't add hot filling to the pastry as it will make it mushy.

Cover the meat with a pastry lid then cover the top of the basin with waxed paper and then a pudding cloth. Secure the pudding cloth with string and gather any excess cloth over the top.

Steam the pudding for 2 hours.

Serve the pudding with the rest of the gravy (reheated separately), boiled potatoes and fresh peas or scarlet runner beans.

Servings: 6 - 8

Personal note

Tastes vary but for me the pastry at the bottom of the bowl has just about the most wonderful flavour you can imagine. Pour as much gravy as you can into the pudding as you serve. This way it has a chance to soak in and flavour the crust.

~~~

INSTANT POT STEAMED PUDDINGS

I love steamed puddings, in fact steak and kidney pudding is probably my most favorite meal of all. And my wife and I are now mostly vegetarian. I'm not worried about the suet but we do try to avoid eating meat most of the time.

One of the drawbacks to eating a steamed pudding is that they are a bit of a pain to cook. You have to keep a close eye on the water level in case you run out or overflow the basin.

The Instant Pot eliminates this drawback and makes cooking suet puddings very easy. They are still not diet food but they certainly make for an occasional treat and are sure to be a hit with your dinner party guest who have probably never tried one before.

To make things easy for you I am repeating most of the recipes in this book but with Instant pot directions.

Instant Pot Spotted Dick

There are many recipes around for Spotted Dick and some of them suggest you make this recipe in a basin, like other steamed puddings. However, that is NOT a traditional Spotted Dick.

This recipe is for a traditional Spotted Dick cooked in a non-traditional way - in an Instant Pot! And that's the only way this recipe differs from the traditional recipe.

Ingredients

    1 recipe sweet suet pastry (see Page 192)

Choose Filling #1

    ¾ cup (115g) currants
    1 small cooking apple, peeled, cored and diced
    ⅓ cup (60g) brown sugar
    ½ large lemon, zest only

or Choose Filling #2

    ¼ cup (40g) currants
    ¼ cup (40g) craisins (dried cranberries)
    ¼ cup (30g) walnuts
    ¼ cup (40g) dried mixed fruit
    ⅓ cup (60g) brown sugar, packed

or Create Your Filling

It's okay to experiment. As long as you keep the quantities about the same you can mix up the filling ingredients. For example, I used raisins instead of currants, chopped almonds instead of walnuts, some chopped candied peel instead of the dried mix fruit ... you get the idea.

Method

In a medium bowl, mix all the filling ingredients together making sure that the brown sugar is well distributed throughout the fruit and nuts. Set aside.

On a lightly floured surface, roll out the sweet suet pastry to form a rectangle approximately 6½ to 7 inches (16.5 to 17.5 cm) by 10 to 11 inches (25 to 28 cm).

Evenly distribute the filling over the pastry and press the filling lightly into the pastry.

Roll up the pastry, as tightly as possible, from the smaller end. For example, start from the edge that is 6½ to 7 inches (16.5 to 17.5 cm) wide so when you are finished you have a Spotted Dick that is 6½ to 7 inches (16.5 to 17.5 cm) long.

Seal the ends and the seam by pinching them together.

Wrap the Spotted Dick well in 2 or 3 layers of aluminum foil and twist the ends to seal.

Place the trivet in the inner liner and pour in 2 cups (480 mL) of boiling water.

Carefully place the foil-wrapped pudding on the trivet.

Close and lock the lid of the Instant Pot, ensuring the Pressure Valve is in the Sealing position.

Select the Steam function and set the cooking time for 45 minutes.

Once cooking time is complete allow for a complete Natural Pressure Release (Wait for the float valve to drop on it's own. This can take up to 45 minutes.)

Remove the completed Spotted Dick from the Instant Pot and allow to cool on a wire rack for 5-10 minutes.

Carefully remove the aluminum foil and slice into serving portions.

Serve with Tate & Lyle's Golden Syrup or Bird's custard.

Instant Pot Apple and Blackberry Pudding

Ingredients

1 recipe sweet suet pastry (see Page 192)

Filling

2 large cooking apples, cored, peel and sliced
1½ cups (190g) blackberries
⅓ cup (65g) sugar

Method

Roll out the sweet suet pastry and line a 1½ pint (700 mL) pudding basin (note: make sure the pudding basin will fit properly in your Instant Pot) with three-quarters of the pastry, reserving one-quarter for the lid.

In a medium bowl, toss together the apple slices, blackberries and sugar. Ladle the fruit and sugar mixture into the pastry-lined pudding basin.

Wet the edges of the pastry lid and then pinch the edges to seal the lid.

Cover the top of the pudding basin with parchment paper or aluminum foil and a pudding cloth. Tie the pudding cloth securely with string and gather any excess pudding cloth over the top of the basin. Note: The pudding cloth is optional, however, you need to make sure that no water gets into the basin while it's steaming. I like to use a pudding cloth because that's the way I've always done it. And, it makes it easier to get the pudding into and out of the pot.

Place the trivet in the stainless steel liner of the Instant Pot.

Add approximately 6 cups (1.4 L) of boiling water to the inner pot (This worked perfect for the basin I used in a 6-quart Instant Pot. The goal is to have the water be about 1" (2.5 cm) below the rim of the pudding basin. Adjust the amount of boiling water to suit your pot and basin.)

Gently lower the prepared pudding basin onto the trivet. Check the water level in relation to the pudding basin and adjust if necessary.

Close and lock the lid of the Instant Pot, ensuring the Pressure Valve is in the Sealing position.

Select the Steam function and set the cooking time for 90 minutes.

Once cooking time is complete allow for a complete Natural Pressure Release (Wait for the float valve to drop on it's own. This can take up to 45 minutes.)

Remove the completed pudding from the Instant Pot and carefully remove the pudding cloth and parchment paper or aluminum foil.

Allow the pudding to cool for 10-15 minutes.

Invert on a serving dish, if desired.

Serve with Bird's custard, heavy cream or ice cream.

Instant Pot Carrot-Raisin Pudding

Ingredients

   2 medium carrots, coarsely grated
   2 medium apples, peeled, cored and finely chopped
   1 medium potato, peeled and finely chopped
   1 cup (125g) suet, chopped (see Page 186 for alternatives)
   1 cup (200g) sugar
   ⅓ cup (80 mL) orange juice
   1 egg, beaten
   1 teaspoon (5 mL) vanilla
   1½ cups (180g) all purpose flour
   1½ teaspoons (7.5 mL) baking soda
   1 teaspoon (5 mL) cinnamon
   1 teaspoon (5 mL) nutmeg, freshly grated
   ½ teaspoon (2.5 mL) ground cloves
   ½ teaspoon (2.5 mL) salt
   1 cup (175g) dates, chopped
   1 cup (150g) raisins

Method

Grease a 2 pint (950 mL) pudding basin (note: make sure the pudding basin will fit properly in your Instant Pot).

In a large bowl, combine the carrots, apples, potato and suet. Mix well.

In a large measuring cup, combine the sugar, orange juice, egg, and vanilla. Mix well and stir into the carrot mixture.

In a medium bowl, combine the flour, baking soda, cinnamon, nutmeg, cloves, and salt. Mix well and stir into the carrot mixture.

Fold the dates and raisins into the carrot mixture.

Pour the batter into the greased pudding basin.

Cover the top of the pudding basin with parchment paper or aluminum foil and a pudding cloth. Tie the pudding cloth securely with string and gather any excess pudding cloth over the top of the basin. Note: The pudding cloth is optional, however, you need to make sure that no water gets into the basin while it's steaming. I like to use a pudding cloth because that's the way I've always done it. And, it makes it easier to get the pudding into and out of the pot.

Place the trivet in the stainless steel liner of the Instant Pot.

Add approximately 6 cups (1.4 L) of boiling water to the inner pot (This worked perfect for the basin I used in a 6-quart Instant Pot. The goal is to have the water be about 1" (2.5 cm) below the rim of the pudding basin. Adjust the amount of boiling water to suit your pot and basin.)

Gently lower the prepared pudding basin onto the trivet. Check the water level in relation to the pudding basin and adjust if necessary.

Close and lock the lid of the Instant Pot, ensuring the Pressure Valve is in the Sealing position.

Select the Steam function and set the cooking time for 120 minutes.

Once cooking time is complete allow for a complete Natural Pressure Release (Wait for the float valve to drop on it's own. This can take up to 45 minutes.)

Remove the completed pudding from the Instant Pot and carefully remove the pudding cloth and parchment paper or aluminum foil.

Allow the pudding to cool for 10-15 minutes.

Invert on a serving dish, if desired.

Serve with Bird's custard, heavy cream or ice cream.

Instant Pot Christmas Plum Pudding

This recipe makes a lot - enough for 4 to 6 steamed puddings depending on the size of basin (bowl) you choose to use - 1½ or 2 pint (700 or 900 mL). You'll need to cook each one individually in the Instant Pot.

Ingredients

    1¼ cups (150g) all purpose flour
    ½ teaspoon (2.5 mL) baking soda
    1 teaspoon (5 mL) salt
    1¼ cups (190g) Sultana raisins
    1¼ cups (190g) seedless raisins
    1 cup (150g) currants
    1 cup (75g) mixed peel, chopped
    1 cup (95g) maraschino cherries
    1 cup (110g) blanched almonds, chopped
    2 tablespoons (15g) all purpose flour
    ½ cup (115g) butter
    1¼ cups (225g) brown sugar, firmly packed
    4 eggs, beaten
    2 tablespoons (30 mL) molasses
    1½ cups (135g) dry bread crumbs
    ½ cup (120 mL) brandy
    1 teaspoon (5 mL) cinnamon
    ½ teaspoon (2.5 mL) nutmeg
    ½ teaspoon (2.5 mL) ground cloves
    1½ cups (185g) suet, finely chopped (see Page 186 for alternatives)
    ⅔ cup (160 mL) milk

Method

In a medium bowl or measuring cup, combine the flour, baking soda and salt. Set aside.

In a medium bowl, mix together the raisins, currants, peel, cherries, nuts and 2 tablespoons (15g) of flour. Toss well so that the flour coats all the other ingredients. Set aside.

In a large bowl cream together the butter and brown sugar until light and fluffy.

Beat the eggs well and add to the butter and sugar mixture. Then add the molasses, bread crumbs, brandy, spices and suet. Mix well.

Add in the floured fruit and nut mixture and mix well.

Add the flour, baking soda and salt mixture alternately with the milk and mix well.

Grease the pudding molds well and fill about 2/3rds full as the puddings will rise.

Cover the top of the pudding basin with parchment paper or aluminum foil and a pudding cloth. Tie the pudding cloth securely with string and gather any excess pudding cloth over the top of the basin.

> Note: The pudding cloth is optional, however, you need to make sure that no water gets into the basin while it's steaming. I like to use a pudding cloth because that's the way I've always done it. And, it makes it easier to get the pudding into and out of the pot.

Place the trivet in the stainless steel liner of the Instant Pot.

Add approximately 6 cups (1.4 L) of boiling water to the inner pot (This worked perfect for the basin I used in a 6-quart Instant Pot. The goal is to have the water be about 1" (2.5 cm) below the rim of the pudding basin. Adjust the amount of boiling water to suit your pot and basin.)

Gently lower the prepared pudding basin onto the trivet.

Check the water level in relation to the pudding basin and adjust if necessary.

Close and lock the lid of the Instant Pot, ensuring the Pressure Valve is in the Sealing position.

Select the Steam function and set the cooking time for 45 minutes.

Once cooking time is complete allow for a complete Natural Pressure Release (Wait for the float valve to drop on it's own. This can take up to 45 minutes.)

Remove the completed pudding from the Instant Pot and carefully remove the pudding cloth and parchment paper or aluminum foil.

Allow the pudding to cool for 10-15 minutes.

You can turn the pudding out at this point and allow it to continue cooling while you start the next on in your instant pot.

Tip: If you have more than one basin, you can be preparing the next one while the previous one is cooking.

Serve with a brandy or rum sauce which you can light just before bringing to the table. The flame may be difficult to see unless you turn out the lights.

Tip: The pudding can be reheated by steaming for about 8 to 10 minutes in the Instant Pot. Follow the directions given above and reduce the cooking time to 10 minutes.

Tip: These puddings will freeze well. Wrap in two layers of waxed paper and then in aluminum foil. Allow to thaw at room temperature when you remove them from the freezer.

Instant Pot Figgy Pudding

Ingredients

¾ cup (95g) suet (see Page 186 for alternatives)
¾ cup (135g) brown sugar, packed
3 eggs
¼ cup (60 mL) cream sherry
1 cup (150g) figs, chopped
¼ cup (60 mL) molasses
1 teaspoon (5 mL) ground cinnamon
1½ cups (135g) dried bread crumbs
1 teaspoon (5 mL) vanilla

Method

Generously grease a 2 pint (950 mL) pudding basin and then coat with white sugar.

In a large bowl, combine the suet and brown sugar and mix well.

Add the eggs, vanilla and molasses and beat until well mixed.

Add the dried bread crumbs and cinnamon and mix until combined.

Add the cream sherry and mix just enough to make sure the sherry is well incorporated into the mixture.

Fold in the chopped figs.

> Note: If you are using dried figs, rehydrate them by putting them in a small saucepan covered with water. Bring them to a boil, reduce heat and allow them to simmer for about 15 minutes. Pour off the excess liquid, allow the figs to cool and then coarsely chop them.

Pour the completed batter into the prepared pudding basin.

Cover the top of the pudding basin with parchment paper or aluminum foil and a pudding cloth. Tie the pudding cloth securely with string and gather any excess pudding cloth over the top of the basin. Note: The pudding cloth is optional, however, you need to make sure that no water gets into the basin while it's steaming. I like to use a pudding cloth because that's the way I've always done it. And, it makes it easier to get the pudding into and out of the pot.

Place the trivet in the stainless steel liner of the Instant Pot.

Add approximately 6 cups (1.4 L) of boiling water to the inner pot (This worked perfect for the basin I used in a 6-quart Instant Pot. The goal is to have the water be about 1" (2.5 cm) below the rim of the pudding basin. Adjust the amount of boiling water to suit your pot and basin.)

Gently lower the prepared pudding basin onto the trivet. Check the water level in relation to the pudding basin and adjust if necessary.

Close and lock the lid of the Instant Pot, ensuring the Pressure Valve is in the Sealing position.

Select the Steam function and set the cooking time for 90 minutes.

Once cooking time is complete allow for a complete Natural Pressure Release (Wait for the float valve to drop on it's own. This can take up to 45 minutes.)

Remove the completed pudding from the Instant Pot and carefully remove the pudding cloth and parchment paper or aluminum foil.

Allow the pudding to cool for 10-15 minutes.

Invert on a serving dish, if desired.

Serve with Bird's custard, heavy cream or ice cream.

INSTANT POT GINGER PUDDING

INGREDIENTS

1 cup (120g) all purpose flour
1½ teaspoons (7.5 mL) ground ginger
¼ teaspoon (1.25 mL) baking soda
½ cup (120 mL) milk
2 tablespoons (30 mL) Tate & Lyle's Golden Syrup
2 tablespoons (30 mL) preserved ginger, chopped
1 egg
1½ cups (135g) bread crumbs
1 tablespoon (15 mL) brown sugar
1½ cups (190g) <u>suet</u> (see Page 186 for alternatives)

METHOD

In a small bowl, combine the flour, ground ginger and baking soda. Mix well and set aside.

In a small saucepan, heat the milk just to the simmering point, remove from heat and add the golden syrup and the beaten egg. Mix well.

> *Note: golden corn syrup may be substituted if you cannot get Tate & Lyle's Golden Syrup*

Stir in the bread crumbs, sugar, suet and chopped, preserved ginger. Add the flour mixture and stir to combine everything well.

Pour the completed mixture into a well greased 2 pint (950 mL) pudding basin.

Cover the top of the pudding basin with parchment paper or aluminum foil and a pudding cloth. Tie the pudding cloth securely with string and gather any excess pudding cloth over the top of the basin. Note: The pudding cloth is optional, however, you need to make sure that no water gets into the basin while it's steaming. I like to use a pudding cloth because that's the way I've always done it. And, it makes it easier to get the pudding into and out of the pot.

Place the trivet in the stainless steel liner of the Instant Pot.

Add approximately 6 cups (1.4 L) of boiling water to the inner pot (This worked perfect for the basin I used in a 6-quart Instant Pot. The goal is to have the water be about 1" (2.5 cm) below the rim of the pudding basin. Adjust the amount of boiling water to suit your pot and basin.)

Gently lower the prepared pudding basin onto the trivet. Check the water level in relation to the pudding basin and adjust if necessary.

Close and lock the lid of the Instant Pot, ensuring the Pressure Valve is in the Sealing position.

Select the Steam function and set the cooking time for 60 minutes.

Once cooking time is complete allow for a complete Natural Pressure Release (Wait for the float valve to drop on it's own. This can take up to 45 minutes or more.)

Remove the completed pudding from the Instant Pot and carefully remove the pudding cloth and parchment paper or aluminum foil.

Allow the pudding to cool for 10-15 minutes.

Invert on a serving dish, if desired.

Serve with Bird's custard, heavy cream or ice cream.

INSTANT POT JAM ROLY-POLY

INGREDIENTS

1 recipe sweet suet pastry (see Page 192)

5 - 6 tablespoons (75 - 90 mL) jam of your choice

METHOD

On a lightly floured surface, roll out the suet pastry to create a rectangle approximately 6½ to 7 inches (16.5 to 17.5 cm) by 10 to 11 inches (25 to 28 cm). (It needs to be sized to fit into the inner liner of your Instant Pot.)

Spread the rolled dough with the jam of your choice. The traditional choices are often raspberry or strawberry jam.

Spread the jam to about ½ an inch (1.25 cm) away from the edges.

Use some cold water to slightly wet the edges of the pastry. Then, roll up the pastry, from the shorter edge and seal the edges and seam.

Wrap the roly-poly well in 2 or 3 layers of aluminum foil and twist the ends to seal.

Place the trivet in the inner liner and pour in 2 cups (480 mL) of boiling water.

Carefully place the foil-wrapped pudding on the trivet.

Close and lock the lid of the Instant Pot, ensuring the Pressure Valve is in the Sealing position.

Select the Steam function and set the cooking time for 45 minutes.

Once cooking time is complete allow for a complete Natural Pressure Release (Wait for the float valve to drop on it's own. This can take up to 45 minutes.)

Remove the completed Roly-Poly from the Instant Pot and allow to cool on a wire rack for 5-10 minutes.

Carefully remove the aluminum foil and slice into serving portions.

Serve with Bird's custard, heavy cream or ice cream.

Instant Pot Leicestershire Pudding

Ingredients

1½ cups (225g) raisins, seedless
1 cup (120g) all purpose flour
¾ cup (95g) suet, chopped (see Page 186 for alternatives)
2 eggs, beaten
1 teaspoon (5 mL) grated lemon peel
1 teaspoon (5 mL) nutmeg, freshly grated
2 tablespoons (30 mL) brandy
milk

Method

Grease a 1½ pint (700 mL) pudding basin.

In a large bowl, combine the raisins, flour and suet and mix well. Mix together the raisins, flour and suet in a bowl.

Add the beaten eggs, lemon peel, nutmeg and brandy. Mix well.

Knead in enough milk to produce a firm dough and transfer the mixture into the greased pudding basin.

Cover the top of the pudding basin with parchment paper or aluminum foil and a pudding cloth. Tie the pudding cloth securely with string and gather any excess pudding cloth over the top of the basin. Note: The pudding cloth is optional, however, you need to make sure that no water gets into the basin while it's steaming. I like to use a pudding cloth because that's the way I've always done it. And, it makes it easier to get the pudding into and out of the pot.

Place the trivet in the stainless steel liner of the Instant Pot.

Add approximately 6 cups (1.4 L) of boiling water to the inner pot (This worked perfect for the basin I used in a 6-quart Instant Pot. The goal is to have the water be about 1" (2.5 cm) below the rim of the pudding basin. Adjust the amount of boiling water to suit your pot and basin.)

Gently lower the prepared pudding basin onto the trivet. Check the water level in relation to the pudding basin and adjust if necessary.

Close and lock the lid of the Instant Pot, ensuring the Pressure Valve is in the Sealing position.

Select the Steam function and set the cooking time for 120 minutes.

Once cooking time is complete allow for a complete Natural Pressure Release (Wait for the float valve to drop on it's own. This can take up to 45 minutes.)

Remove the completed pudding from the Instant Pot and carefully remove the pudding cloth and parchment paper or aluminum foil.

Allow the pudding to cool for 10-15 minutes.

Invert on a serving dish, if desired.

Serve with Bird's custard, heavy cream or ice cream.

INSTANT POT LEMONY SUSSEX POND PUDDING

INGREDIENTS

1 recipe sweet suet pastry (see Page 192)
zest of 1 lemon
½ cup (45g) breadcrumbs
Filling
¾ cup (170g) cold butter, cut into small cubes
¾ cup (135g) brown sugar
1 large whole lemon, (this is a 2nd lemon with the skin intact)

METHOD

When making the sweet suet pastry for this recipe, add the zest of one lemon and the breadcrumbs.

Grease a 1½ quart (1.5 L) pudding basin.

Roll out the sweet suet pastry and line the pudding basin with the pastry. Reserve enough pastry to make a lid for after you have filled the pudding.

Put the lemon on a hard surface and roll it with your hand several times. This will help to release the juice. Prick the lemon all over with a fork or toothpick.

Add half the sugar, butter to the pastry-lined basin and place the whole lemon on top.

Place the remaining sugar and butter around the edge of the lemon.

Wet the edges of the suet pastry lid and place on top. Pinch the edges to seal.

Cover the top of the pudding basin with parchment paper or aluminum foil and a pudding cloth. Tie the pudding cloth securely with string and gather any excess pudding cloth over the top of the basin. Note: The pudding cloth is optional, however, you need to make sure that no water gets into the basin while it's steaming. I like to use a pudding cloth because that's the way I've always done it. And, it makes it easier to get the pudding into and out of the pot.

Place the trivet in the stainless steel liner of the Instant Pot.

Add approximately 6 cups (1.4 L) of boiling water to the inner pot (This worked perfect for the basin I used in a 6-quart Instant Pot. The goal is to have the water be about 1" (2.5 cm) below the rim of the pudding basin. Adjust the amount of boiling water to suit your pot and basin.)

Gently lower the prepared pudding basin onto the trivet. Check the water level in relation to the pudding basin and adjust if necessary.

Close and lock the lid of the Instant Pot, ensuring the Pressure Valve is in the Sealing position.

Select the Steam function and set the cooking time for 90 minutes.

Once cooking time is complete allow for a complete Natural Pressure Release (Wait for the float valve to drop on it's own. This can take up to 45 minutes.)

Remove the completed pudding from the Instant Pot and carefully remove the pudding cloth and parchment paper or aluminum foil.

Allow the pudding to cool for 10-15 minutes.

Invert on a serving dish, if desired.

Serve with Bird's custard, heavy cream or ice cream.

INSTANT POT MIDDLESEX POND PUDDING

INGREDIENTS

1 recipe <u>sweet suet pastry</u> (see Page 192)
zest of ½ orange
½ cup (45g) breadcrumbs

Filling
1 small lemon, thinly sliced
1 small lime, thinly sliced
1 small orange, thinly sliced
2 tablespoons (15g) all purpose flour
¾ cup (135g) brown sugar
½ cup (120g) cold butter, cut into small cubes

METHOD

Grease a 1½ quart (700 mL) pudding basin.

When making the sweet suet pastry for this recipe, add the orange zest and the breadcrumbs.

Roll out the sweet suet pastry and line the pudding basin with the pastry. Reserve enough pastry to make a lid for after you have filled the pudding.

In a medium bowl toss the lemon, lime and orange slices with the 2 tablespoons (15g) of all purpose flour.

To make the filling, create layers starting with 2 tablespoons (25g) of the brown sugar, 3 or 4 cubes of butter and a few slices of lemon, lime and orange. Continue with these layers until you've used up all of the filling ingredients.

Wet the edges of the suet pastry lid and place on top. Pinch the edges to seal.

Cover the top of the pudding basin with parchment paper or aluminum foil and a pudding cloth. Tie the pudding cloth securely with string and gather any excess pudding cloth over the top of the basin. Note: The pudding cloth is optional, however, you need to make sure that no water gets into the basin while it's steaming. I like to use a pudding cloth because that's the way I've always done it. And, it makes it easier to get the pudding into and out of the pot.

Place the trivet in the stainless steel liner of the Instant Pot.

Add approximately 6 cups (1.4 L) of boiling water to the inner pot (This worked perfect for the basin I used in a 6-quart Instant Pot. The goal is to have the water be about 1" (2.5 cm) below the rim of the pudding basin. Adjust the amount of boiling water to suit your pot and basin.)

Gently lower the prepared pudding basin onto the trivet. Check the water level in relation to the pudding basin and adjust if necessary.

Close and lock the lid of the Instant Pot, ensuring the Pressure Valve is in the Sealing position.

Select the Steam function and set the cooking time for 90 minutes.

Once cooking time is complete allow for a complete Natural Pressure Release (Wait for the float valve to drop on it's own. This can take up to 45 minutes.)

Remove the completed pudding from the Instant Pot and carefully remove the pudding cloth and parchment paper or aluminum foil.

Allow the pudding to cool for 10-15 minutes.

Invert on a serving dish, if desired.

Serve with Bird's custard, heavy cream or ice cream.

Instant Pot Treacle Pudding

Ingredients

¼ cup (60 mL) dark treacle, substitute molasses if you can't find treacle
¼ cup (60 mL) Tate & Lyle's golden syrup, substitute corn syrup if you can't find Tate & Lyle's
¼ teaspoon (1.25 mL) cinnamon
2 cups (240g) all purpose flour
3 teaspoons (15 mL) baking powder
1 cup (125g) suet, finely chopped (see Page 186 for alternatives)
⅓ cup (60g) brown sugar
⅓ cup (65g) white sugar
⅔ cup (160 mL) milk
2 eggs, beaten

Method

Grease a 1½ pint (700 mL) pudding basin.

Note: make sure to grease the basin well or the treacle might stick.

Pour the treacle and golden syrup into the base of the pudding basin.

In a medium bowl combine the flour, cinnamon and baking powder and mix well. Cut in the suet with a pastry blender until the mixture resembles a coarse meal.

Add both the white and brown sugar to the flour mixture and stir well.

In a medium bowl, combine the milk and beaten eggs.

Slowly pour the egg mixture into the flour mixture and stir until all ingredients are well combined and make a soft, sticky dough.

Carefully spoon the dough into the pudding basin being careful not to disturb the treacle too much.

Cover the top of the pudding basin with parchment paper or aluminum foil and a pudding cloth. Tie the pudding cloth securely with string and gather any excess pudding cloth over the top of the basin. Note: The pudding cloth is optional, however, you need to make sure that no water gets into the basin while it's steaming. I like to use a pudding cloth because that's the way I've always done it. And, it makes it easier to get the pudding into and out of the pot.

Place the trivet in the stainless steel liner of the Instant Pot.

Add approximately 6 cups (1.4 L) of boiling water to the inner pot (This worked perfect for the basin I used in a 6-quart Instant Pot. The goal is to have the water be about 1" (2.5 cm) below the rim of the pudding basin. Adjust the amount of boiling water to suit your pot and basin.)

Gently lower the prepared pudding basin onto the trivet. Check the water level in relation to the pudding basin and adjust if necessary.

Close and lock the lid of the Instant Pot, ensuring the Pressure Valve is in the Sealing position.

Select the Steam function and set the cooking time for 60 minutes.

Once cooking time is complete allow for a complete Natural Pressure Release (Wait for the float valve to drop on it's own. This can take up to 45 minutes.)

Remove the completed pudding from the Instant Pot and carefully remove the pudding cloth and parchment paper or aluminum foil.

Allow the pudding to cool on a wire rack for 5 minutes and then invert the pudding on a serving plate, allowing the treacle to dribble down the sides.

Instant Pot Cheese and Leek Suet Pudding

Ingredients
1 recipe <u>savoury suet pastry</u> (see Page 191)
Filling
3 tablespoons (40g) butter
1 pound (450g) leeks
2 tablespoons (15g) all purpose flour
1 cup (100g) sharp cheddar cheese, shredded
¼ cup (60 mL) water
1 teaspoon (5 mL) dried thyme
sea salt, to taste
freshly ground black pepper, to taste

Method

Cut the leeks in half, lengthwise and clean well. Remove the tougher green pieces and slice.

In a large skillet, melt the butter over low heat and add the leeks. Cook for about 10 minutes or until soft. Sprinkle the flour over the leeks, mix well and continue to cook, over low heat, for another 2 minutes.

Slowly add the milk, stirring constantly. Then add the grated cheese and stir well to combine.

When the mixture begins to thicken, remove from heat and stir in the salt and pepper to taste. Set aside and allow the mixture to cool completely.

Once the cheese and leek filling has cooled, grease a 2 pint (950 mL) pudding basin, roll out the suet pastry and line the pudding basin with the pastry. Ladle the filling into the basin and then cover with a pastry lid.

Cover the top of the pudding basin with parchment paper or aluminum foil and a pudding cloth. Tie the pudding cloth securely with string and gather any excess pudding cloth over the top of the basin. Note: The pudding cloth is optional, however, you need to make sure that no water gets into the basin while it's steaming. I like to use a pudding cloth because that's the way I've always done it. And, it makes it easier to get the pudding into and out of the pot.

Place the trivet in the stainless steel liner of the Instant Pot.

Add approximately 6 cups (1.4 L) of boiling water to the inner pot (This worked perfect for the basin I used in a 6-quart Instant Pot. The goal is to have the water be about 1" (2.5 cm) below the rim of the pudding basin. Adjust the amount of boiling water to suit your pot and basin.)

Gently lower the prepared pudding basin onto the trivet. Check the water level in relation to the pudding basin and adjust if necessary.

Close and lock the lid of the Instant Pot, ensuring the Pressure Valve is in the Sealing position.

Select the Steam function and set the cooking time for 120 minutes.

Once cooking time is complete allow for a complete Natural Pressure Release (Wait for the float valve to drop on it's own. This can take up to 45 minutes.)

Remove the completed pudding from the Instant Pot and carefully remove the pudding cloth and parchment paper or aluminum foil.

Allow the pudding to cool on a wire rack for 5-10 minutes and serve.

Instant Pot Ham and Leek Suet Pudding

Ingredients

1 recipe savoury <u>suet</u> pastry (see Page 191)

Filling

12 ounces (340g) cooked ham
1 leek
1½ tablespoons (25g) butter
1½ tablespoons (11g) all purpose flour
1 cup (240 mL) chicken stock
2 sprigs fresh thyme
pepper, to taste

Method

Cut the cooked ham into small cubes. Wash the leek well and remove the tough green top of the leek. Then cut the leek into thin slices.

In a medium saucepan, melt the butter over medium heat and cook the leek slices until tender. Sprinkle the flour over the leeks and stir well.

Slowly add the hot chicken stock, stirring constantly. Continue stirring, over medium heat, until the mixture comes to a boil and begins to thicken.

Reduce heat and add the thyme, cream and ham.

Stir well and simmer for about 5 minutes.

Remove from heat and set aside to cool.

Once the ham and leek filling has cooled, grease a 2 pint (950 mL) pudding basin, roll out the suet pastry and line the pudding basin with the pastry. Ladle the filling into the basin and then cover with a pastry lid.

Cover the top of the pudding basin with parchment paper or aluminum foil and a pudding cloth. Tie the pudding cloth securely with string and gather any excess pudding cloth over the top of the basin. Note: The pudding cloth is optional, however, you need to make sure that no water gets into the basin while it's steaming. I like to use a pudding cloth because that's the way I've always done it. And, it makes it easier to get the pudding into and out of the pot.

Place the trivet in the stainless steel liner of the Instant Pot.

Add approximately 6 cups (1.4 L) of boiling water to the inner pot (This worked perfect for the basin I used in a 6-quart Instant Pot. The goal is to have the water be about 1" (2.5 cm) below the rim of the pudding basin. Adjust the amount of boiling water to suit your pot and basin.)

Gently lower the prepared pudding basin onto the trivet. Check the water level in relation to the pudding basin and adjust if necessary.

Close and lock the lid of the Instant Pot, ensuring the Pressure Valve is in the Sealing position.

Select the Steam function and set the cooking time for 60 minutes.

Once cooking time is complete allow for a complete Natural Pressure Release (Wait for the float valve to drop on it's own. This can take up to 45 minutes.)

Remove the completed pudding from the Instant Pot and carefully remove the pudding cloth and parchment paper or aluminum foil.

Allow the pudding to cool for 10-15 minutes.

Invert on a serving dish, if desired.

Instant Pot Steak and Kidney Pudding

Making The Filling

The filling of a steak and kidney pudding is actually a steak and kidney stew. The Instant Pot excels at stew and with this recipe you will be sure to make the best beef stew you have ever tasted. Save what won't fit in your pudding basin to add to the pudding as you serve or freeze it and serve another day as stew.

Ingredients

    3 pounds (1.5 Kg) blade or top sirloin roast, cut into
    ¾ - 1 inch (2 - 2.5 cm) cubes
    1 large onion, cut in bite size pieces
    3 - 4 large carrots, cut into 1 inch (2.5 cm) pieces
    1 tablespoon (15 mL) Bovril™
    1 teaspoon (5 mL) salt, or to taste
    Stock to just cover
    3 ounces (85g) beef kidney, cut into 6 pieces (optional but recommended)
    2 teaspoons (10 mL) cornstarch (or sufficient)

Method

Dust the beef and kidney with unbleached all purpose flour.

Press the Sauté key on the Instant Pot and add the beef and kidney to the stainless steel inner pot, stirring vigorously to prevent the meat from sticking.

When the meat is seared, pour in just enough stock to cover the meat.

Don't add too much liquid as you'll dilute the taste

Add the carrots, onions, Bovril™ and salt.

Close the lid and turn the vent to Sealing

Click the Meat/Stew button add set the time to 30 minutes.

When the time is up Quick release to vent the steam

Mix the cornstarch with just enough water to make it liquid and stir it into the stew. If the stew doesn't thicken you may have to turn on Sauté for a few minutes to bring to simmer while stirring.

The gravy should have the consistency of cooking oil.

Pudding Ingredients

    1 recipe savoury suet pastry (see Page 191)

3 - 4 cups (700 - 900 mL) of the Steak & Kidney filling from the previous page.

¼ cup (60 mL) of the gravy from the stew

METHOD

Grease a 2 pint (950 mL) pudding basin.

Roll out the suet pastry, using ¾ of the pastry for the lining and ¼ for lid.

Line the pudding basin with the pastry and gently ladle the filling into the basin.

> *Use a slotted spoon to avoid putting too much liquid in the pudding which will make the pastry mushy.*
>
> *Make sure the filling is cold or at least cool.*

The basin should be almost full with the drained filling.

Add ¼ cup (60 mL) of the reserved gravy to the filling.

Carefully add the pastry lid and pinch all around the edge to seal it.

Cover the top of the pudding with parchment paper or aluminum foil and a pudding cloth.

Tie the pudding cloth securely with string and gather any excess pudding cloth over the top of the basin.

> *Note: The pudding cloth is optional, however, you need to make sure that no water gets into the basin while it's steaming. I like to use a pudding cloth because that's the way I've always done it. And, it makes it easier to get the pudding into and out of the pot.*

Place the trivet in the stainless steel liner of the Instant Pot.

Add approximately 6 cups (1.4 L) of boiling water to the inner pot (This worked for the basin I used in a 6 quart (6 litre) Instant Pot.

> *The goal is to have the water be about 1" (2.5 cm) below the rim of the pudding basin. Adjust the amount of boiling water to suit your pot and basin.)*

Gently lower the prepared pudding basin onto the trivet. Check the water level in relation to the pudding basin and adjust if necessary.

Close and lock the lid of the Instant Pot, ensuring the Pressure Valve is in the Sealing position.

Select the Steam function and set the cooking time for 45 minutes.

Once cooking time is complete allow for a complete Natural Pressure Release (Wait for the float valve to drop on it's own. This can take up to 45 minutes.)

Remove the completed pudding from the Instant Pot and carefully remove the pudding cloth and parchment paper or aluminum foil.

Allow the pudding to cool for 5 - 10 minutes.

> *Note: This pudding should be served directly from the basin, not turned out onto a plate.*

Serve the pudding with the rest of the gravy (reheated separately), boiled potatoes and fresh peas or scarlet runner beans.

Extra Special Bonus
Mom's Green Tomato Chutney

As a special thanks for buying this 10 volume set I'm including mom's recipe for green tomato chutney.

At the end of summer, as the days started to get colder it was time to think about canning and preserving the fruits and vegetables we still had in the garden. So this was something we made once a year after dad had harvested all the tomatoes that were going to ripen for the season.

We usually made enough to last all year and enjoyed it mostly with meat and cheese. You can use it as a side or add it to sandwiches and hamburgers.

Ingredients

2 - 2½ pounds (approximately 1 Kg) green tomatoes, washed, cored and thinly sliced

7 - 8 ounces (200-225g) onions, halved and thinly sliced

Coarse sea salt

2 pounds (900g) apples (I used Macintosh), washed, cored and chopped

Note: you can peel the apples if you like, but I didn't

6 ounces (170g) brown sugar

½ teaspoon (2.5 mL) turmeric

2 cups (480 mL) malt vinegar

8 ounces (225g) raisins

1½ ounces (45g) pickling spice, tied securely in cheesecloth

Method

The Night Before
1. Combine the sliced green tomatoes and onions in a large glass or ceramic bowl and sprinkle with approximate 3 tablespoons (45 mL) coarse sea salt. Toss slightly.
2. Cover with plastic wrap and allow to sit overnight.
3. The next morning, drain off any liquid and thoroughly rinse and drain the onions and tomatoes.

Spicing The Vinegar
4. Pour the vinegar into a large enamel or aluminum saucepan. Add the pickling spice and boil for 15 minutes.
5. Strain the vinegar through a sieve to remove the spice.
6. Alternatively tie the pickling spice in cheesecloth to make it easier to remove.

Making The Chutney

7. Core and slice the apples and stew in a very little water until just soft.
8. Put everything, except the apples, in a large saucepan with the vinegar, bring to a simmer and stew gently for 1 hour, stirring frequently.
9. Add the apples, stir in well and continue simmering for another hour or until thick.
10. Add more vinegar if you find it gets too thick as you are cooking.
11. Fill approximately six 2-cup (500 mL) sterile canning jars.
12. All the jars to cool to room temperature and then refrigerate or freeze for later use.

Mom's Green Tomato Chutney
Instant Pot Version

When Mom made chutney it used to take up most of the day. This Instant Pot version is just as tasty, and a lot quicker to make.

Ingredients

2 - 2½ pounds (approximately 1 Kg) green tomatoes, washed, cored and thinly sliced
7 - 8 ounces (200-225g) onions, halved and thinly sliced
Coarse sea salt
2 pounds (900g) apples (I used Macintosh), washed, cored and chopped
Note: you can peel the apples if you like, but I didn't
6 ounces (170g) brown sugar
½ teaspoon (2.5 mL) turmeric
2 cups (480 mL) malt vinegar
8 ounces (225g) raisins
1½ ounces (45g) pickling spice, tied securely in cheesecloth

Method

The Night Before
1. Combine the green tomatoes and onions in a large glass or ceramic bowl and sprinkle with approximate 3 tablespoons (45 mL) coarse sea salt. Toss slightly.
2. Cover with plastic wrap and allow to sit overnight.
3. The next morning, drain off any liquid and thoroughly rinse and drain the onions and tomatoes.

Making The Chutney
4. Combine all the ingredients, with the exception of the pickling spice, in the Instant Pot and stir well.
5. Make a small well in the middle of the ingredients and place the cheesecloth-wrapped pickling spice in the well, as close to the bottom as possible.
6. Close and lock the lid, ensuring that the valve is in the Sealing position.
7. Select Manual mode and set cooking time for 5 minutes.
8. Once cooking time is complete, allow a full Natural Pressure Release (this can take more than 20 minutes).
9. Once the pin has dropped (happens when the pressure is totally released), carefully open and remove the lid.
10. Find and remove the cheesecloth-wrapped pickling spice.
11. Stir well.
12. Carefully remove the Instant Pot's inner liner and place on a trivet to allow the chutney to cool.
13. Once the chutney has cooled, package in glass jars and refrigerate or freeze.

BONUS ~ Claim Your Free Book

Thank you for buying this book! As a bonus we would like to give you another one absolutely free - No Strings Attached

You can choose any of the books in our catalog as your bonus. Just use this link or scan the QR code below -

https://fun.geezerguides.com/freebook

Please Review

As independent publishers, we rely on reviews and word-of-mouth recommendations to get the word out about our books.

If you've enjoyed this book, please consider leaving a review at the website you purchased it from

If You're Not Satisfied

We aspire to the highest standards with all our books. If, for some reason, you're not satisfied, please let us know and we will try to make it right. You can always return the book for a full refund but we hope you will reserve that as a last option.

About The Author

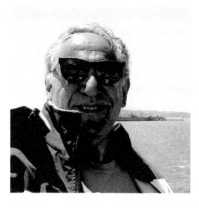

Geoff Wells was born in a small town outside London, England just after the 2nd World War. He left home at sixteen and emigrated to Canada, settling in the Toronto area of Southern Ontario. He had many jobs and interests early in life from real estate sales to helicopter pilot to restaurant owner. When the personal computer era began he finally settled down and became a computer programmer until he took early retirement.

Now, as an author, he has written several popular series including: Authentic English Recipes, Reluctant Vegetarians and Terra Novian Reports, to name a few. He and his wife (and oft times co-author), Vicky, have been married since 1988 and divide their time between Ontario, Canada and the island of Eleuthera in The Bahamas.

Find all of Geoff's books at

https://ebooks.geezerguides.com

Follow Geoff on social media

 https://facebook.com/AuthorGeoffWells/

 geoffwells@ebooks.geezerguides.com

About Our Cookbooks

Quality

We are passionate about producing quality cookbooks. You'll never find "cut and pasted" recipes in any of our books.

Consistency

We endeavor to create consistent methods for both ingredients and instructions. In most of our recipes, the ingredients will be listed in the order in which they are used. We also try to make sure that the instructions make sense, are clear and are arranged in a logical order.

Only Quality Ingredients

To ensure that all of our recipes turn out exactly right, we call for only fresh, quality ingredients. You'll never find "ingredients" such as cake mixes, artificial sweeteners, artificial egg replacements, or any pre-packaged items. Ingredients, to us, are items in their natural (or as close to natural as possible), singular form: eggs, milk, cream, flour, salt, sugar, butter, coconut oil, vanilla extract, etc.

English Speaking Authors

We write all our books ourselves and never outsource them or scrape content from the Internet.

Found an Error?

Although we do our best to make sure everything is accurate and complete, mistakes happen.

If you've found an error - a missing ingredient, an incorrect measurement, a temperature that's wrong, etc. - please let us know so we can correct it.

Just e-mail us at oops@geezerguides.com and we'll make any necessary corrections.

Published by Geezer Guides

When you see *Published by Geezer Guides* on any book, you can be confident that you are purchasing a quality product.

About Geezer Guides

Geezer Guides is a small independent publisher that only publishes original manuscripts. We will never sell you something that has just been copied from the Internet. All our books are properly formatted with a clickable table of contents.

Other Books You May Like

You can find our complete catalog at

https://ebooks.geezerguides.com

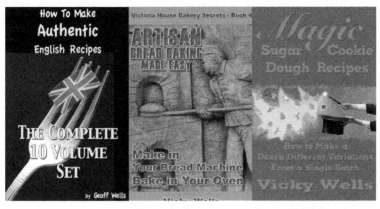

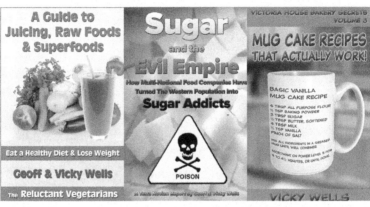

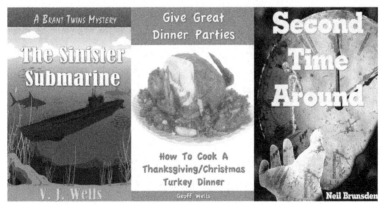

Plus Many More

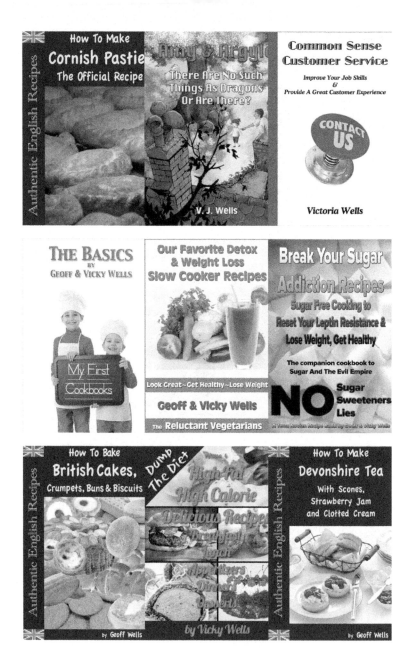

Plus Many More

Made in the USA
Las Vegas, NV
20 January 2021

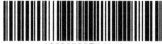